William H. Clarke

The People's Horse, Cattle, Sheep and Swine Doctor

containing concise descriptions of the diseases of the respective animals, with the

exact doses of medicine for each

William H. Clarke

The People's Horse, Cattle, Sheep and Swine Doctor
containing concise descriptions of the diseases of the respective animals, with the exact doses of medicine for each

ISBN/EAN: 9783337235574

Printed in Europe, USA, Canada, Australia, Japan

Cover: Foto ©Andreas Hilbeck / pixelio.de

More available books at **www.hansebooks.com**

THE

PEOPLE'S
HORSE, CATTLE, SHEEP, AND SWINE
DOCTOR:

CONTAINING, IN FOUR PARTS,
CLEAR AND CONCISE DESCRIPTIONS OF THE DISEASES OF THE
RESPECTIVE ANIMALS, WITH THE EXACT DOSES
OF MEDICINE FOR EACH.

EDITED BY

WILLIAM H. CLARKE.

ILLUSTRATED.

NEW YORK:
M. T. RICHARDSON, PUBLISHER.
1892.

COPYRIGHT, 1891.

BY M. T. RICHARDSON.

THE BEN-FRANKLIN PRESS,
45 TO 51 ROSE ST.,
NEW YORK.

PREFACE.

The title page of this work explains its nature, scope, and character so perfectly that little else need be said on the subject. It is compiled from the highest authorities and the latest editions of their respective works. For example, the parts entitled "Medicines and their Doses" and "Medicines and their Classes" are based, or chiefly based, on the seventh edition of Dun's "Veterinary Medicines." Prof. Percivall's works, from which numerous extracts have been made, are getting old, it is true; but as his words are often quoted by all modern veterinary authors, no apology is needed for the extracts from that source in this work. The illustrations, numbering, in the aggregate, 232, are the best of their kind, and are taken from here and there. Many are from Mayhew and Armitage.

One of the drawbacks of most veterinary books is the confusion of nomenclature. This is an almost necessary fault of this volume, for if several of the different names by which some diseases are known were not given, how could the unprofessional reader recognize them? For example, on page 225 is the following: "Carbuncular fever (anthrax), also called Texas fever, splenic fever, trembles, charbon, blain, &c." Page 238: "Hoven (tympanites), also known as hove, hoove, blown, dew-blown, fog-sickness, &c." Page 322: "Swine plague or swine anthrax, also known as hog cholera, red soldier, blue sickness, measles, erysipelas, intestinal fever, typhoid fever, &c." The using of the word 'thrush' to indicate both disease of the foot and the mouth is certainly inexcusable confusion. (See pages 196, 238, 296.) It is like using the word 'fang' to indicate the *root* as well as the crown of a tooth. These and similar defects, in veterinary as well as other works, will probably pass away in the course of time.

As a rule, where practicable, a plain English word has been used to name a disease, the technical name being given in a parenthesis. Where not practicable, the technical name is explained as in the following examples: "Ecthyma (boil-like eruptions)." "Herpes (creeping, spreading)." "Erythema (red, rose-colored)." Scores of other parenthetical explanations are made here and there throughout the work.

The two descriptions of 'Measles' (pages 316 and 328) appear to be inharmonious. The first, based on Gresswell, refers to the well known febrile skin disease; the second, based on Armitage, refers to measle worms. In quoting from different authors, there is sure to be more or less confusion and a few apparent contradictions.

Some useful information is contained in a note on page 13—namely, the measurement of medicines in ordinary utensils. An important addition to the note, especially to farmers, is the fact that an average sized grain of wheat weighs one-half grain—apothecaries' weight.

New York, July, 1891.

INDEX.

NOTE.—As the medicines are alphabetically arranged on pages 13 to 29, they are not indexed; nor are their classes—pages 30 to 37.

ABORTION, cattle 290, sheep 314.
Abscess of scrotum, horse 127.
Abscess, serous, horse 66.
Abuse, self, horse 127.
Actinomycosis (known in the past as cancerous tongue) cattle 228.
Acute indigestion, horse 97.
Acute pulmonary congestion, cattle 263.
Albuminous urine, horse 116, ox 270.
Amaurosis or glass eye, horse 139.
Amputation of the penis, horse 126.
Anæmia or lack of blood, cattle 234.
Anæmic palpitation, cattle 255.
Anthrax (carbuncular or Texas fever) cattle 225, sheep 308, swine 322.
Aphtha or thrush (of mouth) cattle 238, sheep 296.
Apoplexy, cattle 266, swine 324.

BALDNESS, horse 168, cattle 280.
Barrenness, mare 64.
Bees, hornets, &c. stings of, 192.
Belly hernia, horse 59.
Birth, a natural, calf 293.
Bitters, definition and use of (note) 39.
Black Leg or Black Quarter, cattle 227.
Black Water, cattle 270.
Bleeding from lungs, horse 90, cattle 263.
Bleeding from nostrils, horse 76, cattle 258.

Bloody urine, horse 117, cattle 270.
Blue Disease, cattle 255.
Boils, how to treat, cattle 279.
Bog Spavin, horse 197.
Bone brittleness, horse 68, cattle 233.
Bone Spavin, horse 196.
Bots, horse 100, cattle 285, sheep 318.
Broken-Wind, horse 92.
Bronchitis, horse 82, cattle 259.
Bronchitis, chronic, horse 85, ox 260.
Bronchitis, parasitic, cattle 260.
Bronchocele or Goiter, horse 78, cattle 234.
Bruise of the sole, horse 188.
Bruises, general, 188.
Brushing or Interfering, horse 186.
Burns and Scalds, 181.

CANCEROUS TUMOR OF VULVA, mare 126.
Canker in horse's foot, 194.
Capped Elbow, Hock, and Knee, 209.
Carbuncle, cattle 280, sheep 297.
Cataract of horse's eye, 138.
Cataract, green, horse 139.
Catarrh, malignant, ox 231, sheep 300.
Catarrh, simple, horse 70, cattle 258, swine 332.
Cattle Plague, 228.
Cerebro-spinal fever, horse 48.
Choking, horse 155, cattle 239.
Colic, flatulent, horse 104, cattle 245.
Colic, simple, cattle 245,

INDEX.

Colic, spasmodic, horse 102.
Colt Ill (strangles) 42.
Confined (unprotrudable) penis, horse 126.
Congestion of the kidneys, cattle 271.
Congestion of the liver, horse 133.
Congestive Pneumonia, horse 80.
Constipation, horse 110, cattle 246, swine 331.
Consumption, horse 91, cattle 225.
Contagious Pleuro-pneumonia, ox 223.
Corns, horse 200.
Cough, horse 75.
Cow-pox, 229.
Cracked Heel, horse 173.
Crib-biting, horse 144.
Curb, horse 200.

DELIRIUM, cattle 264.
Dental instruments, 145 to 151; the names of same, 152.
Diabetes, horse 63, cattle, 234, 270.
Diaphragm, spasm and rupture of, horse 94.
Diarrhœa, horse 107, cattle 246, sheep 307, swine 332.
Diphtheria, horse 49, cattle 230.
Dislocations, horse 193.
Distention of the rectum, cattle 251.
Dizziness or staggers, horse 55.
Dropsies, horse 64, 65, 66, 127, cattle 250, 280.
Dysentery, horse 108, ox 247, sheep 307.
Dyspepsia, horse 99.
Dysuria (painful urination) cattle 272.

EARS, sheep's, keep clean, 320.
Ecthyma (skin disease) horse 162, ox 279, sheep 298.
Eczema (skin disease) horse 160, ox 275, sheep 297.

Elephantiasis (thick skin) horse 164, ox 278.
Embolism (plugging a vessel) 257.
Engorgement and inflammation of the rumen or first stomach, ox 241.
Engorgement of the omasum or third stomach, ox 240.
Enlargement of kidneys, horse 120.
Enlargement of the lachrymal (eye) caruncle, horse 141.
Epilepsy or fits, ox 265, swine 325.
Equine (horse) syphilis, 121.
Esophagus or throat, stricture, rupture, and opening of, horse 154 155.
Erysipelas, horse 45, cattle 276.
Erythema (skin disease) horse 157, ox 274, sheep 297.
Eyelid, laceration of, horse 180.
Eyes, injuries of, horse 180.

FARDEL-BOUND, cattle 240.
False Quarter, horse 191.
Farcy-Glanders, horse 67.
Fever, brain and spinal cord (cerebrospinal meningitis) horse 48, ox 269.
Fever, acute or inflammatory, horse 39.
Fever, carbuncular or Texas, ox 225, sheep 308.
Fever, catarrhal (influenza) horse 40.
Fever, diphtheritic, horse 49.
Fever, horse-pox, 49.
Fever, low or typhoid, horse 40.
Fever, milk (parturient apoplexy) cow 268.
Fever, purple, horse 47, ox 235.
Fever, pus (strangles or colt-ill) 42.
Fever, scarlet, cattle, 235.
Fever, simple or continued, horse 39.
Fistula, horse 59.
Fistula in the withers, horse 61.
Fistula of the anus, horse 62.

INDEX.

Fistulous Parotid Duct, horse 62.
Flatulent Colic, horse 104, cattle 245.
Flatulent stomach (colic) horse 101.
Flukes, rot of liver caused by, 305.
Flyblow, horse 68.
Foot and Mouth Disease, ox 224.
Foot-Rot, sheep 303.
Foreign bodies in the heart, ox 257.
Fractures, horse 192, cattle 287.
Frost Bite, horse 189.
Foul in the Foot, cattle 286.
Founder, horse 201, cattle 286.

GAD-FLIES, horse 100, cattle 286.
Garget, cattle 289.
Glanders-Farcy, horse 67.
Glass-Eye, horse 139.
Goiter, horse 78, cattle 234.
Gid (sturdy, turnsick, &c.) sheep, 309.
Grass and Stomach Staggers, horse 97, cattle 240.
Grease (skin disease) horse 166.
Green Cataract, horse 139.
Greasiness of the skin, horse 176.

HEART, palpitation of, horse 130.
Heart, various disorders of, horse 130.
Hernia (rupture) horse 58, 59, ox 252.
Herpes (skin disease) horse 161, cattle 276.
Horn Tumor of horse's foot, 208.
Horse-Pox, 49.
Hidebound, horse 173.
Hoven (swelling) ox 238, sheep 317.
Hoose or Husk (worms in throat and bronchial tubes of sheep) 310.
Hydrothorax (water in chest) horse 88.
Hysteria, mare 126.

IMPERFORATE ANUS, cattle 251.
Indigestion, acute, horse 97.

Indigestion, chronic (dyspepsia) horse 99, cattle 245.
Inflamed lymphatics, horse 186.
Inflamed vein, horse 183.
Inflammation of the bladder, horse 119, cattle 273.
Inflammation of the bowels, horse 105, cattle 248.
Inflammation of the brain, horse 48, cattle 264.
Inflammation of the heart, cattle 256, 257
Inflammation of the kidneys, horse 115, cattle 271.
Inflammation of the liver, horse 132, cattle 253.
Inflammation of the lungs (pneumonia) horse 79, ox 261, swine 333.
Inflammation of the mouth, horse 153.
Inflammation of the penis, horse 123.
Inflammation of the pericardium, horse 129, cattle 255.
Inflammation of the peritoneum, cattle 249.
Inflammation of the stomach, horse 96.
Inflammation of the testicles, horse 126.
Inflammation of the tongue, horse 153.
Inflammation of the urethra, horse 123.
Inflammation of the vagina, mare 124.
Inflammation of the womb, mare 125.
Inflammatory pneumonia, horse 80.
Inflation (under skin) cattle 280,
Influenza (catarrhal fever or pink eye) horse 40.
Inguinal (groin) and scrotal hernia or rupture, horse 58.
Injured eyes, horse 180.
Injuries of mouth, tongue, jaws, &c. horse 131,

Interfering or Brushing, horse 186.
Intestinal and stomach concretions (stones) horse 111.
Intussusception or Introsusception, horse 113, cattle 252.
Inversion and protrusion of the bladder, horse 120, cattle 273.

JAUNDICE OR YELLOWS, horse 133, cattle 253.
Joint-Ill, sheep, 312.

KIDNEYS, congestion of, cattle 271.
Kidneys, cysts in, horse 120.
Kidneys, enlargement of, horse 120.
Kidneys, inflammation of, horse 115, cattle 271.

LACERATED KNEE, horse 184.
Lambing or Milk Fever, sheep, 313.
Lampas, horse 153.
Lice, horse 168, cattle 284.
Lichen and Prurigo (skin diseases) horse 159, cattle 278.
Lip, tumor of, horse 154.
Liver, concretions, congestion, rupture, and hydatid tumors of, horse 133; inflammation of, horse 132, cattle 253.
Lock-Jaw, horse 53, with note; cattle 234, sheep 318.
Louping-Ill or Trembling, sheep 314.
Lymphangitis (weed or swelled legs) horse 56.

MALIGNANT CATARRH, ox 231, sheep 300.
Mallenders and Sallenders, horse 202.
Mange, horse 168, cattle 281, sheep 301, swine 334.
'Mark,' the, horse 215, 221.
Measles, sheep 316, swine 328.

Medicines, how to measure them in ordinary utensils (note) 13.
Megrims (vertigo, dizziness, &c.) horse 55, cattle 265.
Milk Fever, cattle 268, sheep 313.
Moon-Blindness, horse 136.
Muir-Ill, cattle 270.

NÆVUS (skin spots of various kinds, often having an erectile character; they may be single or multiple, are more or less pulsating, have a deep purple color, an irregular, flattened appearance, and resemble warts; remedy—absorption, cauterization, adhesive inflammation, excision, or ligature) cattle 280.
Nasal Gleet, horse 73.
Nasal Polypus, horse 77.
Navel Hernia, horse 59.
Navel Ill or Navel Pocking, sheep 312.
Nettle-Rash or Surfeit, horse 158, ox 277.
Non-secretion of Milk, ewe 320.

OBSTRUCTIONS IN THE TEATS, ox 293.
Ophthalmia or Moon-Blindness, horse 136, sheep 319.
Open Knee and other joints, horse 184.
Opening the throat or œsophagus, horse 155.
Opening the windpipe, horse 44.
Osteoporosis (hardening) horse 68.
Ovaries, diseases of, mare 127.
Overreach and Tread, horse 189.
Ozena or Nasal Gleet, horse 73.

PALPITATION OF THE HEART, horse 130.
Paralysis (paresis, palsy) horse 51, ox 266, swine 333.

INDEX.

Parrot-Mouth, horse 143.
Pemphigus or watery bladders, cattle 279.
Penis, amputation of, horse 126.
Piles, horse 113, cattle 251, swine 330.
Pink-Eye (influenza) horse 40.
Pleurisy, horse 86, cattle 262.
Pleuro-pneumonia, contagious, cattle 223.
Pneumonia, horse 79, cattle 261.
Pneumonia, chronic, horse 82.
Pneumonia, inflammatory, horse 80.
Poisons, a few, with antidotes, cattle 236.
Poll-Evil, horse 60.
Polypus, nasal, horse 77.
Polypus of stomach, horse 101.
Pricked Foot, horse 188.
Protruded Penis, horse 126.
Protrusion of the Anus or Rectum, horse 114, cattle 251, swine 330.
Prurigo and Lichen (skin diseases) horse 159, cattle 278.
Pruritus, horse 165.
Psoriasis (scaly inflammation of skin) horse 163.
Pumice Foot, horse 210.

Quinsy (inflammation of the throat or adjacent parts) swine 333.
Quittor, horse 190.

Rabies or Hydrophobia, horse 50, sheep 318.
Red Water, cattle 270, sheep 319.
Retention of urine, horse 120, cattle 272.
Rheumatism, horse 63, cattle 232, swine 333.
Rickets (soft or pliable bone) horse 69, cattle 233.

Ringbone, horse 203.
Ringworm or Tetter, horse 171, cattle 283.
Ringworm, yellow or honeycomb, horse 171.
Roaring, horse 74.
Rot or Fluke Disease, sheep 305.
Rupture, horse 58, cattle 252, 255.
Ruptured tendons and ligaments, horse 187.
Rupture of blood vessels, cattle 255.
Rupture of diaphragm, horse 94.
Rupture of esophagus or throat, horse 155.
Rupture of stomach, horse 101.

Saddle Galls, horse 182.
Saddle Scald, horse 172.
Salivary Calculi (stones) horse 154.
Sallenders and Mallenders, horse 202.
Sandcrack, horse 209.
Scab or Scabies (mange) horse 168, cattle 281, sheep 301, swine 334.
Scrofula, horse 91, cattle 225.
Scarlet Fever, horse 46, cattle 235.
Scrotal and Inguinal (groin) hernia or rupture, horse 58, swine 332.
Scurf (bran-like scales, with slight redness of skin, but without discharge; chronic, non-contagious, with some itching; good habitat for vermin) cattle 280.
Seedy Toe, horse 205.
Self-Abuse in stallion, 127.
Serous Abscess, horse 66.
Sheep-pox, 299.
Sheep Tick, the, 315.
Shivering or Jinkback, horse 210.
Sidebone, horse 204.
Sitfasts, horse 182.
Softening of spinal cord, cattle 269.
Sore and obstructed teats, cows 290.

Sore lips in calves, lambs, goats, and pigs, 276.
Soreness about anus, horse 174.
Sore Throat or Laryngitis, horse 72, cattle 258.
Spasm of the diaphragm, horse 94.
Spasmodic Colic, horse 102.
Spasms and Convulsions, horse 51.
Speedy-Cut, horse, 186.
Spleen, diseases of, horse 135.
Splint (bony tumor or exostosis) horse 198.
Sprain of muscles, tendons, ligaments, horse 187.
Sprain of the back sinews of the hind legs, horse 204.
Staggers, stomach and grass, horse 97, cattle 240.
Staggers (dizziness or vertigo) horse 55.
Stitches or sutures for wounds, horse 178.
Stomach and Intestinal Concretions (stones) horse 111.
Stomach Staggers, horse 97, cattle 264.
Stomachs of the ox, the four, 242.
Stones urinary, horse 118, cattle 273.
Stones or Calculous Concretions, horse 111, cattle 273.
Strain of loins muscles, horse 186.
Strangles (colt ill or pus fever) horse 42.
Strangury (passage of urine drop by drop) 272.
Stricture of the esophagus or throat, horse 154.
Stringhalt, horse 199, cattle 269.
Sturdy (gid, turnsick, turnside) sheep 309.
Suppression and Retention of urine, horse 120, cattle 272.

Surfeit or Nettle-Rash (skin disease) horse 158, cattle 277.
Sutures (stitches) for wounds, horse 178.
Swelled legs (weed or lymphangitis) horse 56.
Swine Measles, cause of and danger from, 328, 329.
Swine Plague (anthrax, hog cholera, red soldier, blue sickness, measles, &c.) 322.
Syphilis, equine, 121.

TEETH, disorders of, horse 142, cattle 288.
Tendons, wounded, horse 185.
Tetanus or Lock-Jaw, horse 53, with note; cattle 234, sheep 318.
Tetter or Ringworm, horse 171, cattle 283.
Texas Fever (anthrax, carbuncular fever, &c.) cattle 225.
Thorough-pin of the Hock, horse 197.
Thorough-pin of the Knee, horse 198.
Thrush (of foot) horse 196.
Thrush or Aphtha (of mouth) cattle 238, sheep 296.
Torpid liver, draft for, cattle 254.
Tracheotomy or opening the windpipe, horse 44.
Tread and Overreach, horse 189.
Trichina Spiralis or Pork Worms, 326.
Tuberculosis or Consumption, horse 91, cattle 225.
Tumor and Fungus of the Orbit, horse 141.
Tumor of the Elbow, horse 182.
Tumor of the Face, horse 154.
Tumor of the Lip, horse 154.
Tumor of the Thyroid Gland, horse 78.

Turnsick, Turnside, Goggles, Gid, &c. sheep 309.
Twins, cow 293.
Twisted or strangled bowels, horse 112, cattle 252.

URINARY STONES, horse 118, cattle 273.

VEIN, inflamed, horse 183.
Venomous bites and stings, 192.
Vertigo or Dizziness, horse 55.

WARBLE OR BOT-FLY, cattle 285.
Warbles or Grubs, horse 183.
Warbles in ox, 183.
Warts, horse 174, cattle 280.
Water on the Brain, cattle 267.
Watery Eyes, horse 140
Weed or swelled legs, horse 56.
Weed, chronic, horse 164.
Windgalls, horse 205.
Worm in the Eye, horse 140.
Worms, horse 111, cattle 287, sheep 310, 311, swine 326–329.
Wounded Tendons, horse 185.
Wounds, horse 177, cattle 287.

YELLOWS OR JAUNDICE, horse 133, cattle 253.

MEDICINES AND THEIR DOSES.

Acid, Acetic.—Is used externally only.

Acid, Hydrochloric.—Of diluted or medicinal acid horses take ½ to 2 drams* (drachms), cattle 2 to 4 drams, sheep and swine 15 to 20 drops, in 40 or 50 times its bulk of water, often given with bitters and iron.

Acid, Nitric.—Of diluted medicinal acid horses and cattle take 1 to 2 drams, sheep and swine 10 to 20 drops, largely diluted with water; often conjoined with bitters. For external use, a dram in a pint of water is strong enough for all except escharotic (caustic) purposes. An ointment and a paste are also used.

Acid, Nitro-Hydrochloric.—Diluted and in the same doses as nitric acid.

Acid, Sulphuric.—Horses take of the medicinal acids 1 to 2 drams, cattle 2 to 4 drams, sheep ½ to 1 dram, swine 10 to 20 drops, several times a day, freely diluted and often conjoined with aromatics and bitters. As an external astringent, 10 to 20 drops of medicinal acid are mixed with an ounce of water.

Aconite.—Horses, 20 to 30 drops; cattle ½ to 1 dram; sheep and swine, 5 to 10 drops. Fleming's tincture of aconite is about 4 times stronger than most others, and must be used accordingly.

---

* A teaspoon contains 1 fluid dram; a dessert-spoon 2; a table-spoon 1-2 a fluid ounce; a wine glass 2 to 2 1-2 fluid ounces; teacups 5 to 7 fluid ounces; common tumblers from 8 to 10 fluid ounces.

In *apothecaries' weight* 20 grains make 1 scruple, 3 scruples 1 dram, 8 drams 1 ounce; (pound not used except at wholesale, when 16 ounces, avoirdupois, is the standard). In *fluid measure* 60 minims make 1 dram, 8 drams 1 ounce, 16 ounces 1 pint, 2 pints 1 quart, 4 quarts 1 gallon. In England 20 ounces make 1 pint, imperial measure.

Alcohol.—Of rectified spirit, that is, alcohol made from grain, not the kind made from wood, horses take about 1 oz. (ounce), cattle 1 to 3 oz., sheep ½ oz., swine 2 drams. Rectified spirit is also called spirit of wine. Whisky, gin, and brandy are about half the strength of rectified spirit; sherry and port about a third the strength of whisky; ale about half the strength of sherry and port. In critical cases they have to be given at intervals of 1 or 2 hours.

Aloes.—Horses, 2 to 10 drams; cattle, 1 to 2 ounces; sheep, ½ to 1 ounce; swine, 2 to 5 drams, twice a day. For colts allow 5 grains for every week of their age. Aloes purge the blood as well as the bowels.

Alums.—Horses and cattle, 2 to 4 drams; sheep and swine, 20 grains to 2 drams, in ball or solution.

Ammoniæ Liquor Fortior.—Horses, 1 to 2 drams; cattle, 2 to 4 drams; sheep and swine, 1 dram. Liquor ammoniæ and aromatic spirit of ammoniæ, being about half the strength, are given in double doses.

Ammonium Carbonate.—Horses, 2 to 4 drams; cattle, 3 to 6 drams; sheep and swine, 15 to 60 grains, in ball, linseed meal, or gruel. Used cold.

Ammonium Chloride.—In same doses as ammonium carbonate.

Ammonii Acetatis (Liquor).—Horses and cattle, 1 to 4 ounces, given in 5 or 6 parts of water, diluted spirit, or linseed tea. Diluted spirit means half alcohol and half water.

Amyl-Nitrite.—Horses and cattle, 3 to 10 drops. Try small dose first. When given hypodermically, half doses usually suffice. Inhaled, on sugar or in draught, with rectified spirit or ether.

Anise.—Horses, 1 oz.; cattle, 1 to 2 oz.; sheep and swine, 2 to 3 drams, several times daily, powdered. Anise oil, mixed with a little spirit and olive or other mild oil, destroys lice. Linseed, palm, and cod liver are also mild oils. 'A little spirit' means alcohol (in proportion.)

Antimony Tartrate (Tartar Emetic).—When given to horses or cattle for sedative, alterative, or expectorant effects, 1 to 4 drams, 3 or 4 times daily, in ball or solution. As an emetic for swine, 4 to 10 grains.

Areca-Nut.—Horses, 4 to 6 drams, in soup, mucilage, or milk. Also called catechu or betel-nut palm.

Arnica, Tincture.—Horses, 4 drams to 1 ounce; cattle double the quantity, in water, ale, or gruel.

Arsenic.—Horses and cattle, 1 to 6 grains; sheep, 1 to 2 grains. Usually given once a day for 8 or 10 days.

Asafetida.—Horses, 2 to 4 drams; cattle, 1 ounce; sheep, 1 dram, several times daily, in ball or solution.

Atrophine (Sulphate).—Horses and cattle, 1 to 3 drams. Hypodermically, 1-5 or less the quantity. For prompt and marked antispasmodic and anodyne effects, it should be combined with equal parts of morphine.

Belladonna.—Of the dried powdered leaves horses and cattle take about 2 ounces. It is usually made into extracts, succus, or tincture. Of the green extract (British Pharmacopeia process), horses take 1 to 2 drams, cattle 2 to 3 drams, sheep 10 to 20 grains.

Bismuth.—Of the sub-nitrate horses take 1 to 2 drams.

Boric Acid.—Horses and cattle, 3 to 6 drams; colts and calves, 20 to 30 grains.

Bromides.—Horses, 1 to 2 drams, in ball or water.

Broom.—Horses, 1 ounce of the succus (the fluid obtained by pressing plants, flesh, &c.)

Buchu.—Of the leaves horses and cattle take 1 to 4 ounces, in linseed tea or barley water.

Caffeine.—Horses, 10 grains; hypodermically (under the skin), 5 grains.

Calabar Bean.—Horses and cattle, 15 to 30 grains.

Calcium Oxide.—Of quicklime horses and cattle take 1 to 2 drams, sheep 20 to 30 grains. Of lime-water horses and cattle, 4 to 5 ounces; sheep, 2 drams to 1 ounce. Two ounces of lime-water and gentian infusion often check diarrhea in feeble calves; half the dose for sheep. For calves and dogs saccharated lime is used as an antacid and stomachic. It is made by rubbing an ounce of slaked lime with two ounces of sugar, transferring the mixture to a bottle containing a pint of water, shaking, and separating the clear solution with a siphon. It renders the milk conveniently alkaline, without diluting it as the limewater does. Antacids obviate acidity of the stomach.

Calcium Carbonate.—Horses, 1 to 2 oz.; cattle, 2 to 4 oz.; sheep, 2 to 4 drams; swine, 1 to 2 drams, in ball or solution.

Calcium Chlorata.—Horses, 1 to 2 drams; cattle, 2 to 4 drams; sheep, about 1 dram.

Calcium Phosphate.—Horses and cattle, 1 to 2 drams; sheep, 5 to 10 grains, in food.

Calomel.—See 'Mercurous Chloride.'

Camphor.—Horses, 1 to 2 drams; cattle, 2 to 4 drams; sheep and swine, 20 to 40 grains. For external use dissolve in 6 or 8 parts of proof spirit, linseed oil, or oil of turpentine. Proof spirit consists of 5 pints of rectified spirit and 3 pints of water.

Cannabis Indica.—Horses and cattle take the extract in ½ to 1 dram doses. Tincture—horses, 1 to 2 drams; cattle, 2 to 4 drams.

Cantharides.—Horses, 4 to 20 grains; cattle, 10 to 20 grains; sheep and swine, 2 to 8 grains, once or twice a day.

Carbolic Acid.—Horses and cattle, 15 to 40 drops; sheep and swine, 5 to 8 drops, in ball, water, or glycerine and water. Better in fluid.

Cascarilla Bark.—Horses, 2 to 4 drams; cattle, 1 oz.; sheep and swine, 1 to 2 drams, in ball, infusion, or tincture.

Castor Oil.—Horses and cattle, about a pint; sheep and swine, 2 to 4 oz., alone or with gruel, milk, or aromatics.

Catechu.—Horses, 1 to 3 drams; cattle, 2 to 6 drams;

sheep and swine, 1 to 2 drams, 3 or 4 times a day, in mucilage or gruel.

Chamomile Flowers.—Horses and cattle, 1 to 2 oz.; calves, sheep, and swine, 1 dram. Sometimes used as fomentations and poultices.

Charcoal (Carbon).—Horses, 4 drams to 1 oz.; cattle, 1 oz.; sheep and swine, 1 to 3 drams, in gruel or other mucilaginous fluid.

Chloral (Hydrate).—Horses, 2 to 4 drams; cattle, 4 drams to 1 oz.; sheep and swine, $\frac{1}{2}$ to 2 drams, in sirup (syrup), every 2 or 3 hours.

Chlorine is made by heating common salt and manganese black oxide with sulphuric acid. The gas is inhaled or the fresh solution applied in spray for ulcerated or diphtheritic sore throat in horses, and to abate the discharge and fetor in diseases of the facial and frontal sinuses (cavities). Both destroy the mites infesting the air-passages of calves and lambs. The liquor chlori (water charged with chlorine gas) is often introduced into the windpipe. Chlorine is irritant, stimulant, antiseptic (opposed to putrefaction), deodorant, and disinfectant.

Chloroform.—Horses and cattle, 1 to 2 oz.; sheep and swine, 4 drams to 1 oz.; given on blotting paper or sponge for sheep and swine; on sponge or in bag for horses and cattle; put sponge in nostril. The chloroformed horse must have its knees protected with stout caps. Internal dose—horses and cattle, 1 to 2 drams; sheep and swine, 20 to 40 drops, in sirup, mucilage, whisked egg, or weak alcohol, every 2 or 3 hours.

Chloroform, Spirit of.—Horses, 1 oz.; cattle, 2 oz.; sheep and swine, 2 to 6 drams, in water.

Cinchona.—Horses, 2 to 4 drams; cattle, 1 to 2 oz.; sheep and swine, 1 to 4 drams, 2 or 3 times daily for several days, reducing the dose or intermitting for a day or two if nausea occurs. The above doses are for the bark. An infusion is made by digesting for 1 hour, in a covered vessel, 1 part of red bark in No. 40 powder with ¼ part of aromatic sulphuric acid and 20 parts of water; strain. A tincture is made by maceration and percolation of 4 ounces of red bark, No. 40 powder, in 1 pint of proof spirit.

Quinine is made by boiling the bruised cinchona bark with diluted hydrochloric acid, and mixing the filtered solution with lime until it is alkaline, when a precipitate falls; is collected and boiled with alcohol, which dissolves both the quinine and cinchonine. Quinine is obtained from different cinchonas, but chiefly from the yellow, and is the active principle of those valuable drugs. Horses and cattle, 20 grains to 1 dram; sheep and swine, 5 to 20 grains, in ball, pill, or solution, 2 or 3 times daily.

Cinnamon.—Horses 4 drams to 1 oz. of the bark, 20 drops to 1 dram of the oil, on sugar, in sirup, &c.

Cod-Liver Oil.—Horses, 2 oz.; cattle, 2 to 4 oz.; sheep, 1 oz.; swine, 4 drams to 1 oz., twice a day and repeated for weeks, omitting if diarrhea sets in; given in milk, gruel, eggs, &c.

Colchicum (Autumn Crocus or Meadow Saffron).—Horses, ½ to 1 dram; cattle, 1 to 2 drams; sheep, 10 to 25 grains; swine, 2 to 8 grains, powdered and given in salines. Salines contain a salt, or have the properties of a salt.

Copper Sulphate (Blue Vitriol).—Horses, 1 to 2 drams; cattle, 1 to 4 drams; sheep, 20 to 30 grains; swine, 5 to 10 grains, in ball or solution, twice a day.

Creosote.—Horses, 10 to 30 drops; cattle, ½ to 1 dram; sheep, 5 to 15 drops; swine, 2 to 10 drops, in ball or sirup.

Croton Seed and Croton Oil.—Horses, 10 to 12 seeds (3 grains to each seed); cattle, 15 to 20 seeds; sheep, 3 to 4 seeds; swine, 2 to 3 seeds. Of the oil, horses, 15 to 25 drops; cattle, ½ to 2 drams; sheep and swine, 5 to 10 drops.

Corrosive Sublimate.—See 'Mercuric Chloride.'

Curare (A South American arrow poison).—Horses and cattle, ½ to 1 grain. It is more effective if injected intravenously or subcutaneously (into a vein or under the skin).

Digitalis.—(So called because the flower resembles a finger stall; also called Fox Glove.) Of the powdered leaves horses take 10 to 30 grains; cattle, ½ to 1 dram; sheep, 8 to 15 grains; swine, 2 to 10 grains. Of the tincture, horses and cattle, 2 to 4 drams; sheep, 1 dram. The fluid extract made in the United States is nearly 10 times as strong as the B. P. (British Pharmacopeia) tincture. A horse was poisoned by two ounces of the powdered leaves in twelve hours. In some cases six drams have caused death in from twelve to sixteen hours.

Epsom Salt.—See 'Magnesium Sulphate.'

Ergot (of Rye).—As an ecbolic for the mare or cow, ½ to 1 oz.; for sheep and swine, 1 dram, every ½ or 1 hour. Swallow dregs and all. Sometimes 100 lbs. of hay yields 1 lb. of ergot. Ecbolics are used to cause abortion or to hasten parturition. Avoid ergot pastures in grazing.

Ergotin.—Horses and cattle, 15 to 25 grains. When used hypodermically, smaller doses should first be tried.

Ether.—As a stimulant horses take 1 to 2 oz.; cattle, 2 to 3 oz.; sheep and swine, 2 to 4 drams, in cold water, diluted spirit, &c.

Eucalyptus (Blue Gum Tree).—Horses and cattle, 1 dram, in diluted spirit, mucilage, or milk.

Fern Root.—Of the powdered root horses and cattle take ¼ lb.; sheep, 3 to 5 oz. Liquid extract—horses and cattle, 2 to 4 drams; sheep, 1 dram. The extract is less bulky and surer.

Galls.—Of tannic acid horses take 20 grains to 2 drams; cattle, 3 drams; sheep and swine, 15 to 30 grains. Tannic acid is the principle to which oak-bark galls, logwood and many vegetable astringents owe their properties. Galls, tannic and gallic acids differ only in the degree of their action.

Gamboge (A Gum Resin).—Cattle, $\frac{1}{2}$ to 1 oz.; sheep, 20 to 30 grains, given with other purgatives and in solution.

Gentian—Horses, $\frac{1}{2}$ to 1 oz.; cattle, 1 to 2 oz.; sheep, 1 to 3 drams; swine, $\frac{1}{2}$ to 1 dram, 2 or 3 times daily, in ball or infusion.

Ginger.—Horses, 4 drams to 1 oz.; cattle, 1 to 3 oz.; sheep, 1 to 2 drams; swine, $\frac{1}{2}$ to 1 dram, in ball.

Gum Arabic.—Horses and cattle, 2 to 3 oz.; foals, calves, and sheep, 1 oz.

Glycerine, given shortly before meals, is useful in checking undue gastric (stomach) fermentation, acidity, and flatulence, both in calves and dogs. It is the basis of many dressings for blisters, burns, cracked heels, &c.

Hellebore.—Do not use without medical advice. A powdered ounce, with 2 ounces of alum, dissolved in a gallon of hot water, will destroy caterpillars.

Hemlock.—Of the fluid horses and cattle take 2 to 4 oz.; sheep and swine, $\frac{1}{2}$ to 1 oz. Neither the dried leaves nor fruit is reliable.

Henbane (Hyoscyamus Leaves).—(Poison Tobacco, Stinking Nightshade.) Of the tincture horses and cattle take 1 oz. The extract is 6 times as strong as the tincture. Hyoscyamine, usually given as a neutral sulphate, is 100 times more active than the extract. Sometimes used hypodermically. The leaves and seed are the parts used in medicine. Eaten by swine.

Iodine.—Horses, 20 grains to 1 dram; cattle, $\frac{1}{2}$ to $1\frac{1}{2}$ dram; sheep, 15 to 40 grains; swine, 10 to 20 grains, 1 or 2 times daily, 2 hours after eating, for a week or 10 days, omitting for a day or two if necessary.

Ipecac (Ipecacuanha).—Of the powder, as an emetic, swine take 20 to 30 grains, in tepid water, either alone or with $\frac{1}{2}$ to 1 grain of tartar emetic. Some use Dover's powder (1 part each of ipecac and opium and 8 parts of potassium sulphate). Of this expectorant and diaphoretic horses and cattle take 1 to 3 drams; sheep, 30 grains to 1 dram, several times daily. Plenty of diluents; clothe comfortably; atmosphere 60° F. Expectorants induce coughing, hawking, and spitting. Diaphoretics excite perspiration. All watery drinks are diluents.

Iron, Sulphate (Green Vitriol).—Horses, $\frac{1}{2}$ to 2 drams; cattle, 1 to 4 drams; sheep, 10 to 30 grains; swine, 5 to 20. The smaller doses are given as tonics and for the blood, the larger as astringents, 2 or 3 times daily, in ball, solution, or food.

Iron, Iodide.—Same doses as iron sulphate. Avoid overdoses.

Iron, Chloride.—Of the medicinal liquor and tincture horses and cattle take $\frac{1}{2}$ to 1 oz.; sheep, 20 to 30 drops; swine, 10 to 20 drops. Taken at the same intervals and for the same purposes as sulphate of iron, above.

Jaborandi.—Of the fresh leaves, as an infusion, horses and cattle take 2 to 4 drams; sheep and swine, $\frac{1}{2}$ to 1 dram. Pilocarpine nitrate or hydrochlorate (a component part of jaborandi), is used hypodermically in horses and cattle in 1 to 2 grain doses.

Jalap.—As a purgative for swine, 1 to 4 drams, combined with a grain or two of calomel.

Juniper.—Of the fruit as a stomachic horses and cattle take 1 to 3 oz.; sheep, 2 to 4 drams, several times a day, coarsely powdered and mixed with fodder. Of the oil, distilled from the unripe fruit, as a diuretic, horses and cattle take 1 to 2 drams, every 3 hours till water passes freely. Diuretics increase the secretion of urine.

Laudanum.—See 'Opium.'

Lead Acetates.—Horses and cattle, $\frac{1}{2}$ to 1 dram; calves and sheep, 10 to 20 grains; swine, 2 to 4 grains, once or twice a day, in ball or solution. External use— Sugar of lead is used in powder, ointment, or dissolved in 20 to 40 parts of water, with a little vinegar, to increase its solubility. Goulard's extract, diluted with 4 to

6 parts of linseed or olive oil, is a cooling application for blistered or contused surfaces. An equally valuable astringent and anodyne is Goulard's extract, 1 part, vaselin or glycerine, 6 to 8 parts. Equal parts of Goulard's extract and alcohol, diluted with 8 to 10 parts of water, make a useful refrigerant astringent.

Lead Iodide is occasionally prescribed as a gland stimulant, and applied as a dressing for ringworm and indolent tumors. Used as ointment or plaster.

Linseed Oil.—As a purgative horses take $\frac{1}{2}$ to 1 pint; cattle, 1 to 2 pints; sheep and swine, 6 to 12 oz.; shaken up in linseed gruel, milk, &c. For horses and cattle it is sometimes mixed with a well-made bran mash.

Magnesia.—Colts and calves of 3 or 4 months old, take, as an antacid, $\frac{1}{2}$ to 1 dram. It is conjoined with carminatives and given in milk or gruel. Carminatives allay pain.

Magnesium Sulphate (Epsom Salt).—As a purge, given in 10 or 15 parts of water, cattle take 1 to $1\frac{1}{2}$ lb.; calves of 2 or 3 months, 3 to 4 oz.; sheep and swine, 4 to 6 oz. To expedite purgation and prevent nausea and griping, add a dram of ginger to the oz. of salt. One-fifth or one-eighth of these doses are often effectual in removing indigestion, keeping up the action of other cathartics, and as febrifuges and alteratives. On horses, when given alone, it is uncertain. For febrifuge and alterative purposes, in any class of patients, it is conjoined with niter, mineral acids, gentian, and other bitters. Cathartics are either purges or laxatives. Febrifuges are opposed to or abate fever. Alteratives are supposed to produce salutary changes in diseases, but without exciting any sensible evacuation.

Mercurous Chloride (Calomel).—As an alterative and febrifuge horses and cattle take 10 grains to 1 dram; sheep and swine, 5 to 30 grains, usually 2 or 3 times a day, and frequently with equal weight of opium, to prevent too rapid purging. As a purge calomel should be combined thus: For horses—calomel, 1 dram, aloes, 4 drams. Cattle—calomel, 1 to 2 drams, Epsom or common salt, 1 lb., or oil, 1 pint. As a vermifuge (worm destroyer) for horses: Calomel, oil of male shield fern, and aloes, 1 dram each; ginger, 4 drams, in ball, with linseed meal and molasses. As an emetic for dogs or swine: Calomel, 2 to 3 grains; tartar emetic, same; or (in place of tartar emetic) 15 to 20 grains ipecac. Calomel destroys the acari (parasites) of scab and mange, kills lice, abates the itching of eczema and prurigo, removes the scales and heals the cracks of psoriasis, hastens the removal of warts, and is one of the best remedies for thrush in the horse's frog. In the form of ointment, it relieves piles in dogs. It should be used discreetly.

Mercuric Chloride (Corrosive Sublimate).—Horses and cattle, 5 to 8 grains; sheep and large pigs, 1 grain, in water or other simple fluid. For most external uses, a solution is made of 2 to 5 grains to the oz. of water. For itching—corrosive sublimate, 2 grains, prussic acid, 2 drops, water, 1 oz. Ointment—corrosive sublimate, 1 part, fatty matters, 12 to 20 parts, usually the latter; used for skin and parasites.

Mustard.—As a stomachic, carminative, or mild stimulant horses take 4 to 6 drams; cattle, $\frac{1}{2}$ to 1 oz.; sheep and swine, 1 to 2 drams, in pill or electuary (confection.) Large doses act as emetics in dogs, cats, and swine.

Myrrh.—(A brown-red gum-resin, from the coasts of the Red Sea.) Horses and cattle, 2 drams; sheep and swine, $\frac{1}{2}$ to 1 dram, several times daily, in ball, decoction, or tincture; used with other tonics or with aloes.

Nux Vomica (Strychnine).—Of powdered nux vomica horses take $\frac{1}{2}$ to 1 dram; cattle, 1 to 2 drams; sheep, 10 to 40 grains; swine, 10 to 20 grains. The extract is 8 or 10 times as active as the powder. A tincture is sometimes used. Strychnine is more uniform and more readily absorbed than the crude drug, and upward of 50 times more powerful. Horses, 1 to 2 grains; cattle, 2 to 5 grains; sheep, 1-5 to 1 grain. Both forms are usually given twice a day.

Oak Bark.—Horses, 2 to 4 drams; cattle, ½ to 2 oz.; sheep and swine, ½ to 2 drams. It is made with 1 or 2 oz. of bark to a pint of water; given with aromatics and bitters; in dysentery, with opium and starch gruel; in typhoid fever, with camphor and mineral acids.

Olive Oil.—Small doses are occasionally given to horses and other animals to soothe the irritated mucous membrane in chronic catarrh and bronchitis. Bronchitis is inflammation or catarrh of the bronchial (lung) tubes.

Opium.—Of solid opium horses take 1 to 2 drams; cattle, 2 to 4 drams; sheep, 10 to 40 grains; swine, 5 to 20 grains. Of morphine and its salts horses and cattle take 3 to 10 grains; sheep and swine, ½ to 2 grains. For hypodermic injections use the small doses first. Tincture of opium (laudanum)—horses and cattle, 1 to 3 oz.; sheep and swine, 2 to 6 drams.

Pepper, Black.—As a stomachic horses take about 1 dram; cattle, 2 drams; sheep and swine, 10 grains to ¼ dram, in ball, water, alcohol, or gruel.

Peppermint.—Horses and cattle, 20 to 30 drops, on sugar or in alcohol and water.

Pepsin is a preparation of the mucous lining of the fresh and healthy stomach of pigs, sheep, or calves. Colts and calves, 2 to 10 grains, in water, with a few drops of hydrochloric acid.

Petroleum Benzin is used as a vermifuge, killing even tapeworms. Horses take 2 to 4 drams.

Podophyllum.—(May Apple or Mandrake.) For cholagogue (cathartic) or sedative purposes horses and cattle take 1 to 2 drams of the resin (podophyllin), with aloes or calomel, or with niter or Epsom salt. Ginger prevents nausea and griping. Sedatives depress the vital forces.

Potassium Bromide.—Horses and cattle, ½ to 1 oz., every two hours, in water.

Potassium Carbonate and Bicarbonate.—Of either kind horses and cattle take ½ to 1 oz.; sheep and swine, ½ to 1 dram, several times a day, liberally diluted with water. For stimulating gastric secretions they are given half an hour before eating; but in most dyspeptic cases acids are more permanently effectual.

Potassium Chlorate.—(Chlorate of Potash.) Horses, 1 to 4 drams; cattle, 2 to 6 drams; sheep and swine, 20 to 60 grains, 2 or 3 times daily, in ball or solution, alone, or conjoined with bitters, tonics, or stimulants. Most horses will take an ounce a day of their own accord. As a soothing electuary for sore throat, it is conjoined with camphor, belladonna extract, and molasses.

Potassium Iodide.—Horses and cattle, 2 to 6 drams; sheep and swine, 20 to 60 grains, two or three times a day, in ball or solution.

Potassium Nitrate (Niter).—As a diuretic horses take ½ to 1 oz.; cattle, 1 to 2 oz.; sheep, 1 to 2 drams; swine, ½ to 1 dram. For fever ¼ the dose, several times daily.

Potassium Permanganate.—As an alterative and febrifuge horses and cattle take 1 dram, but it is not preferable to either the nitrate or chlorate.

Potassium Sulphide.—Horses and cattle, 1 to 3 drams, for chronic cough, rheumatism, and skin diseases.

Prussic or Hydrocyanic Acid.—Of the B. P. 2 per cent. acid horses and cattle take 20 drops to 1 dram; sheep and swine, 10 to 20 drops, 3 or 4 times daily, in sweetened water.

Quassia Wood.—Of the B. P. infusion (chips, 1 part, cold water, 80 parts, macerated 1 hour) horses and cattle take 2 to 4 oz.; sheep and swine, 4 drams.

Quinine.—See 'Cinchona.'

Rhubarb.—As a stomachic and tonic horses take 1 oz.; cattle, 2 oz.; sheep, 1 dram, several times a day. It is used as powder, infusion, or tincture. Rhubarb, 2 parts, magnesia, 6 parts, ginger, 1 part, all in fine powder and thoroughly mixed, make an excellent stomachic and antacid; doses double those of simple rhubarb. In diarrhea in calves and foals it exerts carminative, laxative and subsequently astringent effects. When the bowels are persistently relaxed, 2 drams each of rhubarb and magnesia, with $\frac{1}{2}$ a dram of opium, may be given night and morning in well-boiled wheat-flour gruel, with 1 or 2 tablespoonfuls of spirits or sweet spirit of niter. One-third or one-half the quantity for lambs. 'Spirits' mean whisky, brandy, gin, rum, &c., as well as alcohol.

Salicylic Acid.—Horses and cattle, 1 to 2 drams; sheep, 10 to 15 grains, every 1 or 2 hours, with an equal quantity of borax to insure solubility; ball or solution.

Savin.—As a destroyer of worms horses and cattle take 3 or 4 drams of the volatile oil, dissolved in any mild fixed oil, or in mucilage. Decoctions and ointments are used externally.

Silver Nitrate.—Horses and cattle, 2 to 5 grains; sheep, 1 to 2 grains; swine, $\frac{1}{2}$ to 1 grain, 2 or 3 times daily; ball.

Sodium Carbonates.—Of the carbonate horses and cattle take 1 to 2 drams; sheep and swine, 10 to 50 grains. The bicarbonate, possessing only about half the strength of the carbonate, is given in double doses; ball or water.

Sodium Sulphate.—As a purgative cattle take 1 to $1\frac{1}{2}$ lb.; sheep, 2 to 4 oz., in ginger and molasses, followed by a liberal supply of chilled water.

Sodium Sulphites and Hyposulphites.—Of the sulphites horses and cattle take $\frac{1}{2}$ to 1 oz.; sheep and swine, $\frac{1}{2}$ to 1 dram. Of the hyposulphites $\frac{1}{4}$ these doses. Take either several times daily, in powder or solution, or with food.

Sodium Chloride (Common Salt.)—As a purgative adult cattle take $\frac{3}{4}$ to 1 lb.; sheep, 1 to 3 oz.

Sodium Chlorata.—Of the B. P. solution (about $2\frac{1}{2}$

per cent. of the available chlorine), horses and cattle take 1 to 2 oz.; sheep and swine, 1 to 2 drams, in water.

Spirit of Nitrous Ether.—As a stimulant and antispasmodic horses take 1 to 3 oz.; cattle, 1 to 4 oz.; sheep, 2 to 4 drams; swine, 1 to 2 drams. Do not mix with other medicines or water till ready to give. Give in cold water or linseed tea. Antispasmodics allay spasms.

Squill.—Horses take ½ dram of the sirup. The acetate and tincture are given in about half the dose of the sirup.

Strophanthus.—Of the tincture (1 part to 20 of rectified spirit) horses take ½ to 1 dram. The seeds are used in Africa as an arrow poison.

Strychnine.—See 'Nux Vomica.'

Sugar.—Of sugar and molasses, as laxatives, horses and cattle take 1 pound; sheep, 3 to 4 oz.; swine, 2 to 3 oz., given, with aromatics and salines, in water, milk, gruel, or mash.

Sulphur.—As a laxative horses take 1 to 4 oz.; cattle, 3 to 6 oz.; sheep and swine, 4 drams to 1 oz. As an alterative ¼ the quantity.

Sulphurous Acid.—Of the B. P. solution horses and cattle take 1 to 2 oz.; sheep and swine, ½ to 1 dram, every 3 or 4 hours, in water or other mild fluid.

Taraxacum (Dandelion Root).—The fresh succus is the best preparation. Horses about 1 oz.

Thymol.—For vesical catarrh horses take 5 to 20 grains. Its chief use is in antiseptic surgery.

Turpentine.—Horses and cattle, 1 to 3 oz.; sheep, 1 to 3 drams; swine, 1 to 2 drams, in milk, oils, eggs, &c. The larger doses are stimulant and antispasmodic; the smaller, frequently repeated, are diuretic and inspissant (thickening).

Turpentine Oil (Spirit).—As a stimulant and antispasmodic horses and cattle take 1 to 2 oz.; as a diuretic ¼ to 1 oz.; as an adjuvant cathartic or vermifuge about 2 oz., combined with aloes in solution, castor or linseed oil, iron salts, quassia, gentian or other bitters. Large cattle take double these doses. Sheep and swine, 1 to 4 drams; given in mild oils, linseed gruel, milk, &c. An adjuvant medicine is introduced into a prescription to aid the operation of the chief ingredient or basis.

Valerian.—Horses and cattle, 2 to 4 oz., several times daily, in powder or infusion, conjoined with ginger, gentian, or camphor, or dissolved in spirit of ammonia.

Veratrum Viridi and Album.—(Green and White Hellebore Rhizome.) Of the powder horses and cattle, $\frac{1}{2}$ to 1 dram; sheep and swine, 20 to 30 grains, every 3 or 4 hours, in ball or dilute alcohol. Used externally in the several forms of powder, watery decoction (improved by a little spirit), and ointment, made with 1 part of veratrum to 8 of vaselin or lard. It is occasionally applied with tar or sulphur dressings.

Verdigris, Blue (Copper Subacetate) is an irritant poison, and is rarely used internally. It is used externally as a caustic, stimulant, astringent, and antiseptic.

Water is a valuable diluent, febrifuge, and evacuant. It should be given moderately cold and at frequent intervals. Except for a few hours previous to great exertion, and when hungry, overheated, and prostrated, healthy horses should not be restricted in their water supply. But it must always be given judiciously, especially to the sick.

Zinc Oxide.—Horses and cattle, 2 to 4 drams, in ball or solution. For external use there are solutions, liniments, ointments, and pastes or powders.

Zinc Sulphate.—As an astringent and tonic for horses and cattle, 1 to 3 drams; sheep, 10 to 20 grains, in solid or fluid state. As an emetic for swine and dogs 8 to 15 grains, in 2 or 3 ounces of water. Externally it is used in powder or solution—30 to 60 parts of water for the latter. Zinc sulphate, $\frac{3}{4}$ oz., lead acetate, 1 oz., water, 1 quart, constitute the well-known 'white lotion.' It is a valuable astringent, sedative, and antiseptic.

The foregoing doses, except where otherwise specified, are for adult animals of medium size. Stallions, bulls, and rams, owing to their larger size, require larger doses. Difference of sex does not materially affect dosage in the lower animals. Doses must be adapted to the age of the patient. It is usually estimated that a 1-year-old colt requires one-third the quantity of any medicine given an adult horse; a 2-year-old, one-half; a 3-year-old, two-thirds. A somewhat similar proportion is applicable to cattle.

Medicines are usually given (1) internally, that is, by the stomach; (2) by inhalation; (3) by absorption through the skin. The latter mode has also three ways of administration—epidermically, by in-rubbing; endermically, by removing the epidermis (skin); hypodermically, by injection into the tissues under the skin. A ready but less prompt or certain substitute for hypodermic injection with a syringe, consists in coating a thread with a strong solution of the medicine to be introduced, and drawing it through the skin. Medicine may be injected into the veins or arteries; but this mode is rare and usually experimental.

MEDICINES AND THEIR CLASSES.

Alkalies are caustic bases, are soluble in water and alcohol, unite with oils and fats to form soap, neutralize and change reddened litmus paper to blue, &c. Potash, soda, ammonia, lime, and magnesia are the chief alkalies.

Alkaloids are usually powerful poisons or active medicines. Those chiefly used are morphine, atrophine, quinine, cocaine, pilocarpine, ergotinine, coniine, nicotine, and spartcine. Alkaloids are salifiable bases, that is, they are capable of combining with an acid to form a salt. They are mostly derived from vegetable plants, in which they are usually the active principle. Alkaloid means a kind or form of alkali.

Alteratives influence the amount and kind of tissue change going on in different organs and cells. Sodium chloride, sulphate, phosphate, acetate, and biborate; potassium nitrate, ammonium chloride and carbonate, and probably all salts excreted by the kidneys, increase tissue change and the quantity of urea excreted. The urea is a component part of the urine.

Anesthetics (Anæsthetics) diminish and absorb sensation. Chloroform, ether, chloral hydrate, nitrous oxide, chloride of olefiant gas, light coal-tar naphtha, &c. Used locally (that is, for certain spots)—cocaine, carbolic acid, and iodoform.

Anaphrodisiacs diminish sexual passion. Ice or cold water locally; potassium iodide and bromide; purgatives, digitalis, and camphor; a spare diet and steady work.

Anhydrotics check perspiration and skin secretion. Belladonna and atrophine, picotoxine, nux vomica, salts of zinc, &c.

Anodynes relieve pain. Opium, morphine, anesthetics in small doses, belladonna, atrophine, chloral, conium, hyoscyamus, stramonium, &c.

Antacids obviate acidity of the stomach. They consist of the alkalies, namely, potash, soda, ammonia; the alkaline earths, lime and magnesia, and their carbonates and bicarbonates, &c. Horses instinctively lick lime-washed walls or eat earth when suffering from acidity of the stomach.

Anthelmintics kill or expel intestinal worms. For bots—green food; a combination of aloes, asafetida, turpentine, and ether. For tapeworms—areca-nut, filixmas, kamala, kousso, pomegranate, turpentine, and chloroform. For round worms—santonin, santonica (wormseed plant). For thread worms—turpentine and essential oils, tannin and tannin-containing substances; santonin, santonica; with injections of common salt, iron chloride, or limewater. For fluke worms—maintain strength by good feeding; common salt and soluble iron salts exert general tonic effects and limited vermicide action; a physic hastens expulsion of the flukes.

Antiperiodics mitigate the severity or prevent the recurrence of certain diseases. Cinchona, quinine, and arsenic are reliable antiperiodics.

Antiphlogistics.—See 'Antipyretics.'

Antipyretics lower the temperature of the body in fever. They embrace cinchona alkaloids, benzoic, carbolic, and salicylic acids, salicylicates, salicin, camphor, eucalyptol, thymol and other essential oils, alcohol, antimonial salts, aconite, digitalis, veratrine, nitrous ether, antipyrin, opium, ipecac, cold bath, wet pack, cold drinks, ice to surface, &c.

Antiseptics arrest putrefaction. Carbolic, nitric, hydrochloric, sulphuric, salicylic, and boric acids, corrosive sublimate, iodine, creosote, zinc and iron chlorides, iodoform, ethereal oils, alcohol, eucalyptus, &c. Antiseptics may yet be discovered capable of checking the multiplication of septic germs in the blood and tissues, as they now do in a wound, or external to the body. (Dun.)

Antispasmodics prevent or remove spasms. Sulphuric ether, valerian, asafetida, musk, castor and aromatic oils, alkaline bromides, salts of silver, zinc, and copper.

Antizymotics not only arrest fermentation, but they destroy the several classes of ferments. Corrosive sublimate, chlorine, iodine, bromine; sulphurous, carbolic, boric, salicylic, and benzoic acids; many metallic solutions; temperatures above 200° F.

Aperients.—See 'Purgatives.'

Aphrodisiacs increase sexual appetite. When there is lack of vigor, the most rational treatment consists in the administration of tonics—iron, strychnine, &c. Cantharides is unsafe.

Astringents contract the tissues with which they come in contact and diminish their secretions. Alum, lime, chalk, salts of the heavier metals, acids, and alcohol, with tannic acid and such tannin-containing substances as oak bark and catechu.

Blisters.—Cantharides, glacial acetic acid, turpentine, strong ammonia, and boiling water. See 'Counter-irritation.'

Carminatives allay pain by causing the expulsion of flatus (gases) from the stomach and intestines. They are closely allied to antispasmodics. Chief among them are the various aromatic oils, with ginger, mustard, peppers, alcohol, ethers, and chloroform. Carbonic acid gas is neutralized by ammonia preparations; sulphureted and carbureted hydrogen gases by solutions of chlorine or lime chloride.

Cataplasms.—See 'Poultices.'

Cathartics.—See 'Purgatives.'

Caustics burn and disorganize the parts to which they are applied, causing sloughing. The most active are called escharotics; they are also called corrosives. They consist of the concentrated mineral acids and alkalies, glacial acetic acid, carbolic acid, chromic acid, antimony chloride, arsenic, bromine, and the soluble salts of the heavy metals.

Charges.—See 'Plasters.'

Cholagogues.—See 'Purgatives.'

Counter-Irritation is irritation of a healthy part to counteract irritation or disease of a contiguous part. Mustard, croton oil, tartar emetic, iodine, mercurial ointment, mercuric iodide, vinegar of cantharides, and water (nearly boiling).

Demulcents soothe, soften, and ensheathe parts; they act mechanically chiefly and resemble emollients. Gums, mucilage, linseed, cotton-wool and collodion, fullers' earth, starch, molasses, gelatin, albumin, fats, oils, glycerine, and milk.

Deodorizers destroy smells. Chlorine, chloride of lime, carbolic, sulphurous, and cresylic acids, iodine dissolved in amyl-hydride, Condy's fluid, McDougall's powder, &c.

Diaphoretics excite perspiration. They are uncertain as a class. They are all indirect agents; some sedative, others excitant, and cannot therefore be used indiscriminately in disease. Ammonia acetate solution, sweet spirit of niter, sulphuric ether, diluted spirits, jaborandi, ipecac, or Dover's powder, warm or vapor baths—100° to 120° F.

Diluents.—All watery drinks are diluents.

Disinfectants destroy the specific poisons of communicable diseases. Chlorine, chlorinated lime, carbolic acid, sulphurous acid, corrosive sublimate solutions, iodine, &c.

Diuretics act on the kidneys and increase their secretions. Digitalis, alcohol, strophanthus, squill, strychnine, caffeine, broom, turpentine, juniper, copaiba, cantharides, nitrites, liquor potassæ, potassium acetate, &c. Ball for horse—$\frac{1}{2}$ oz. each of niter, resin, and soft soap, daily for 4 or 5 days. If it is desirable to increase the solid as well as the watery parts of the urine, add 10 or 15 grains of powdered digitalis. The same ingredients, dissolved in a pint of water, make a diuretic drink for the cow.

Ecbolics expel the contents of the uterus; they cause abortion or hasten birth. Ergot, hydrastis, savin, and thuja. Ergot is the only one is general use.

Emetics cause vomiting. Luke warm water, bitter infusions, solutions of salt, mustard, alum, ammonium carbonate, copper and zinc sulphates; tartar emetic, ipecac, emetine, apomorphine, senega, squill.

Emollients soften, soothe, and relax parts. They resemble 'demulcents' (which see), and include many of the medicines specified in that class. Warmth or moderate heat, generated by fomentations, poultices, lint, flannel, or woolen cloth, and retained by a waterproof covering, are a species of emollient. Fats, oils, lanolin, vaselin, paraffin, with soap and other liniments, are emollients.

Emulsions are soft, smooth, milk-like mixtures of oil or resin, suspended in gum, soap, alkali, or white of egg.

Expectorants aid in removing secretions from the air passages. Those of a depressant type are such as the antimonials, alkalies in small doses, ipecac, lobelia, jaborandi, apomorphine, and potassium iodide. The stimulating are such as the acids, ammonium salts, nux vomica, senega, squill, balsams, terebinthinates, sulphur, sulphur oils, and saccharines (sweets).

Febrifuges.—See 'Antipyretics.'

Fomentations are topical baths. They usually consist of water alone, but vinegar, salines, &c., are sometimes added. They are usually made with a sponge or soft rags, tow, or lint. The temperature ranges from 100°, 110°, 120° F., and upward.

Germicides destroy germs or bacteria. Sodium hydrofluosilicate (recently discovered) is a cheap and safe germicide. (Dun.) Corrosive sublimate, chlorine, chlorinated lime, bromine, iodine, quinine, beberine, &c., are all good germicides, especially corrosive sublimate.

Infusions are made by digesting vegetable substances or drugs in hot water (usually 1 part of drugs to 20 of water) 15 minutes to 2 hours. Avoid boiling.

Lotions (washes) are watery solutions for external use, especially in chronic skin diseases. Strong lotions may be used as counter-irritants. Lotions for the eye are usually called collyria.

Narcotics are soothers as well as stupefiers. Opium, morphine, ether, chloroform, aconite, belladonna, digitalis, hyoscyamus, stramonium, conium, &c.

Plasters usually contain lead oxide, conjoined with resin, wax, soap, fats, tar, or pitch, spread on calico, linen, or leather.

Poultices are made of linseed meal, bran, or oatmeal, stirred into boiling water until the fitting consistence is reached; or of carrots or turnips, either steamed or boiled. Bread and starch make mild porous poultices for abscesses; spent hops for light poultices. Apply in flannel bag or folded flannel.

Purgatives evacuate the bowels. They are usually classified as follows: Laxatives or Aperients—small doses of oil, magnesia, sulphur and molasses, with fruit, roots, and green vegetable food. Simple Purgatives—full doses of oils, aloes, and the various species of rhamnus. Drastic Purgatives—croton oil, colocynth, elaterium, gamboge, and podophyllin. Hydragogues—elaterium, gamboge, croton oil, &c., with large doses of the more active salines. Cholagogues—calomel and other mercurial preparations, aloes, jalap, podophyllin, and euonymin, for bile. Salines —(See 'Salines,' page 36.) Purgatives and other irritants should be used cautiously in the case of the horse. If possible, the animal should be restricted to mash diet or green food for 24 hours previous to taking a purgative.

Refrigerants allay heat and thirst. Water, particles of ice, acidulated drinks, mild mucilaginous fluids, allay thirst and stimulate the secretion of saliva.

Rubefacients cause slight redness of the skin and congestion. Ammonia solutions, mustard, iodine, mild preparations of cantharides, arnica, alcohol, ether, chloroform (if not allowed to evaporate), turpentine and many other volatile oils, with smart friction and moderate heat, such as that from a smoothing iron. The smoothing iron is good for rheumatism and enlarged joints.

Salines contain a salt or have the properties of a salt. They consist of the neutral salts of the alkalies and alkaline earths, such as magnesium sulphate and citrate, sulphate of soda, potassium tartrate and bitartrate, &c. As before said, 'magnesium sulphate,' is simply Epsom salt (commonly called 'salts').

Sedatives lessen the force and frequency of the heart's action. Aconite, veratrum viridi, and the antimonials; also digitalis, lead acetate, opium, ergot, and topical applications.

Sialagogues increase the secretion of saliva. Acids, alkalies, ethers, mustard, ginger; jaborandi, calabar bean, and their alkaloids; mercury, tobacco, iodide of potassium, &c.

Soporifics or Hypnotics induce sleep. Opium, morphine, alcohol hydrate, croton-chloral, hyoscyamus, cannabis, bromides, &c.

Stimulants.—Ammonium and its carbonate, alcoholic solutions, capsicum, nux vomica, ether, chloroform, oil of turpentine and other volatile oils, aromatic oils, camphor, opium and cocaine in small doses, &c.

Styptics are astringents specially used to arrest effusion of blood from injured surfaces or vessels. They are (1) matico, tow, lint, or pressure; (2) most astringents and caustics (which see); (3) ergot, digitalis, ether spray, lead acetate, ice, &c.

Sudorifics.—See 'Diaphoretics.'

Suppurants inflame the deep seated skin tissues and bring pus. Euphorbium, croton oil, tartar emetic, mercury biniodide ointment; also cantharides, mustard and other active blisters, when repeatedly applied to the same spot.

Tonics impart strength. Sulphuric acid, nitric acid, iron, iron and copper sulphates, arsenic, cinchona, quinine, quassia, cocaine, cod-liver oil, gentian, silver nitrate, zinc oxide, buchu, &c. Heart Tonics—digitalis and its alkaloids, casca (doom) and its active principle, erythrophlœin, strophanthus hispidus, squill, caffeine, nux vomica, and strychnine.

Vermicides.—See 'Anthelmintics.'
Vermifuges.—See 'Anthelmintics.'
Vesicants.—See 'Blisters.'

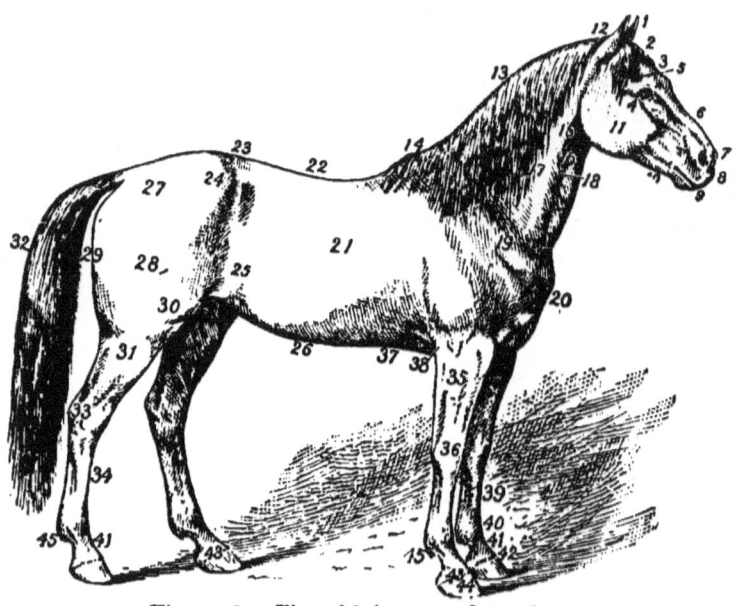

Figure 1. The chief parts of the horse.

1 Ears.
2 Forelock.
3 Forehead.
4 Eye.
5 Eye-pit.
6 Nose.
7 Nostril.
8 Tip of Nose.
9 Lips.
10 Lower Jaw.
11 Cheek.
12 Poll.
13 Mane.
14 Withers.
15 Parotid Gland
16 Throat.
17 Neck.
18 Jugular Vein.
19 Shoulder.
20 Chest.
21 Ribs.
22 Back.
23 Loins.
24 Hip.
25 Flank.
26 Belly.
27 Haunch.
28 Thigh.
29 Buttock.
30 Stifle.
31 Leg.
32 Tail.
33 Hock.
34 Shank or Cannon
35 Arm.   [Bone.
36 Knee.
37 Place for Girth.
38 Elbow.
39 Shank.
40 Bullet.
41 Pastern.
42 Coronet.
43 Foot.
44 Hoof.
45 Fetlock.

PART I.

THE DISEASES OF THE HORSE.

SIMPLE OR CONTINUED FEVER

Is a comparatively mild and benign disease, lasting from two to eight days. It disturbs all or nearly all the chief functions of the body, occurs independently of local inflammation or blood contamination, and is common among horses brought into dealers' stables.

Remedy.—Comfortable box; fresh air and light; quiet. Clothe body; bandage legs; mild laxative. Salines; ammonium acetate solution; potassium chlorate or nitrate; spirit nitrous ether. Mash diet; gruel; diluents; withhold hard, dry food. Alcohol, ether, bitters,* acids; tonic as soon as acute symptoms abate. Catarrh, gastro-intestinal or other special symptoms must receive appropriate treatment. (For doses, see pages 13 to 29.)

ACUTE OR INFLAMMATORY FEVER

Concurs with acute local inflammation.

Remedy.—Aconite; occasional bleeding in early stages in robust subjects. Aperients, salines, laxative injections. Attend to any wounds; remove any causes of irritation.

---

* Bitters are usually spirituous liquors in which bitter herbs or roots have been steeped, such as aloes, cascarilla bark, various cinchona barks, gentian, myrrh, nux vomica, quassia, &c. Combinations of acids and bitters have long been used in dyspepsia, the good effects of the latter being believed to result from their stimulating the movements of the stomach, and from their action on the liver. (Dun.)

Warm clothing, but cool air to breathe. Warm bath or sponging with warm water. Sodium sulphite, sulphocarbolates, resorcin, or other antiseptics and antipyretics. Alcohol and digitalis sustain heart tone. Salicylic acid and salicin in rheumatic fever. Acids and bitters allay thirst and aid digestion. Light, easily digested food; diluents; salines in drinking water. For doses, see pages 13 to 29.

LOW OR TYPHOID FEVER

Occurs in most epizootics in connection with blood contamination, in inflammation of mucous membranes, and in debilitated subjects.

Remedy.—Mild laxatives and injections when required. Salines, acids, bitters, antiseptics. Quinine, especially in intermittent types. Arsenic in malarial cases. Alcohol, ethers, or volatile oils promote excretion and maintain heart action. Turpentine and iron salts for bleeding cases. Suitable clothing; diet; hygiene (preservation of health); sponging; baths. For doses, see pages 13 to 29.

INFLUENZA,

Also called Catarrhal Fever, Pink Eye, &c., is usually epizootic and, comet-like, appears at irregular intervals. Its worst visitation in North America perhaps was that of 1872-73. Little is known of the exact nature of the disease. It differs in form and symptoms as it appears in different localities and at different times. Robertson describes four forms of the disease—(1) simple catarrhal; (2) pulmonary; (3) intestinal catarrhal; (4) rheumatic. Some of these forms may be caused by active living organisms (mites). The disease is very infectious. Severe cases constitute pink eye.

Symptoms.—Simple catarrhal: As before said, they differ, but there are usually shivering fits, more or less loss of appetite, sneezing, coughing; a somewhat dry or staring coat, eyes watery, the conjunctive membrane sometimes being of a clear pink color (pink eye); nasal membrane red and dry; pulse 60 to 70; temperature 104; dullness, debility, &c. These symptoms may steadily increase in severity. Runs its course in about 14 days.

The pulmonary form, which is dangerous, may either follow or be independent of the simple form. It has three

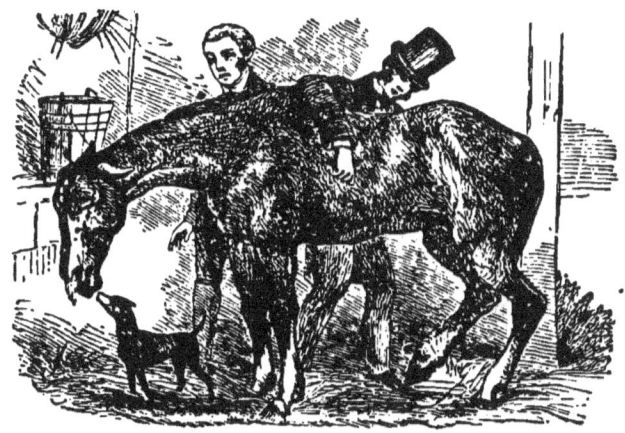

Fig. 2. Confirmed Influenza.

forms—(1) capillary bronchitis; (2) bronchitis with heart disease; (3) pneumonia, or rather pleuro-pneumonia.

The intestinal catarrhal form is sometimes so distinct, and one of its symptoms or complications is so evidently connected with the special functions of the liver, as to cause it to be called bilious fever. The symptoms resemble those of mild colic.

The rheumatic form is usually a sequel to the simple catarrhal. The parts usually affected are the great tendons of the flexor muscles of the foot.

Remedy.—Isolate patient and disinfect the premises. Comfortable box; temperature 60 to 65° F.; pure air. Rugs, hood, bandage legs. Injections, linseed mashes and, if necessary, a laxative for bowels. Liquor ammoniæ acetatis, Epsom salt, and niter for fever. Mash diet, with a little green food, till fever abates; then digestible, concentrated, nutritive food.

Catarrhal symptoms treated by steaming head, medicated inhalations, or sprays. (See 'Catarrh.') Flannels wrung out of hot water and mustard, or other embrocations, to the throat relieve congestion of the upper air passages. Embrocations are fluid remedies for in-rubbing.

Swelling symptoms, treated with salines and antiseptics, require early use of such stimulants as alcohol, ether, oil of turpentine, or ferric chloride solution.

Pneumonic cases: Liquor ammoniæ acetatis, potassium nitrate or chlorate, and camphor. Fomentations to chest; mustard applied, but washed off in 15 or 20 minutes; reapplied if necessary, or injection of Savary's mustard extract. With salines give alcohol and ether, early, but in moderate doses, every three hours.

Gastro-intestinal complications treated in earlier stages by a few doses of gray powder or calomel, conjoined with laxatives; in later stages by nitro-hydrochloric acid. Abdominal pain relieved by chloral and cannabis indica internally, or by morphine hypodermically.

Rheumatic symptoms: Salicylic acid, oil turpentine, diuretic doses of digitalis and salines, with stimulation of affected muscles and joints. Patients, if reduced, require milk, eggs, beef tea, and frequent alcoholic stimulants. (For doses, see pages 13 to 29.)

STRANGLES (PUS FEVER, COLT ILL),

Is a common and well defined disease, but veterinarians are not agreed as to its exact cause or nature. It is attributed by some to a strepto-coccus, which settle on and irritate the nasal membrane. It is peculiar to but not limited to young horses, and seldom occurs but once. The fever (Percivall calls it 'strangles fever') is nearly always followed by an abscess or abscesses in the space between the branches of the lower jaw, involving the adjacent glands. The pus mites, it is said, are liable to be carried to and inflame other glands in the shoulder, groin, or internal organs.

The disease is probably contagious, and is sometimes epizootic. It is well named, for it sometimes causes death by strangulation. Robertson describes two forms of it—"regular or benign," which is easily cured, if not self-curable, and "irregular and malignant," which is dangerous. It is disposed to run a 'regular' course, and should be aided rather than retarded. The tumor, when

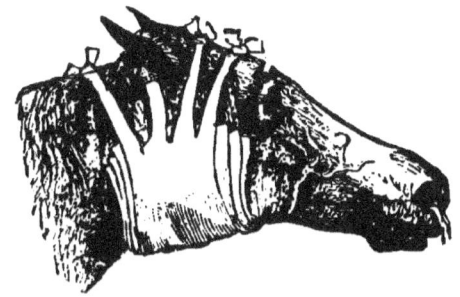

Fig. 3. Poultice and 8-tailed bandage for Strangles.

ripe, may be lanced, or it may be allowed to burst naturally. Its most dangerous sequels are pus fever and purulent and putrid blood poisoning.

Symptoms.—Usually mild catarrhal discharges; dull; cough, pickish appetite, throat sore, interfering with swallowing; head pointed forward; mouth hot and dry; may be cutting the corner incisor teeth or the tushes; if so, make crucial incisions over them; in doubt till tumor appears under the jaw; tumor steadily increases in size, becoming hard, defined, painful.

In the irregular or complicated form there is sometimes a slight swelling at the jaw, but instead of maturing it recedes, and may attack the glands of the head, neck, chest, or even more remote parts, intensifying and multiplying the symptoms.

Remedy.—Good nursing; soft or green food. Perfect sanitary surroundings. Steam head where catarrhal symptoms are troublesome. Fomentations or poultices hasten tardy abscesses. Sodium sulphite and potassium chlorate in the drinking water oppose fever and blood poisoning. Sweet spirit of niter and quinine also for blood poisoning. Cleanse discharging abscess daily with carbolic oil. Isolate; disinfect premises. Milk, eggs, beef tea, with ale or wine if the animal is weak. When at grass, shelter at night. For doses, see pages 13 to 29.

Tracheotomy affords instant relief, and is a safe operation. The incision is made at the point indicated in the annexed cut. Should it be made higher than this,

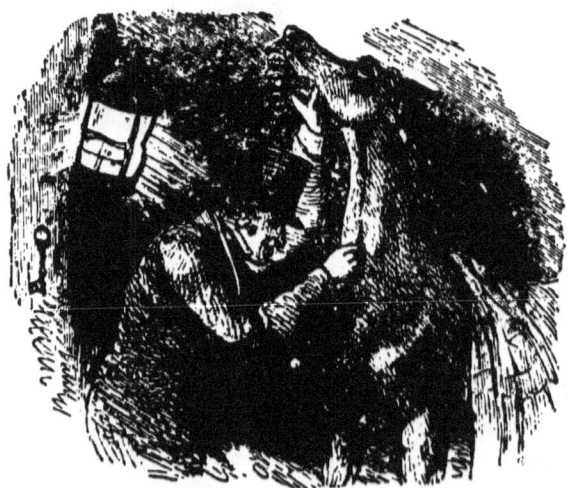

Fig. 4. Performing the operation of Tracheotomy by Lamp Light.

the tube will interfere with the application of a poultice. Provided with a needle and thread, make a longitudinal incision three or four inches in extent down to the windpipe. After the windpipe has been pierced and the animal is in some measure relieved, draw the thread through the part that is to be removed, so that it cannot be drawn inside and thus increase the impediment to breathing. After this, cut out a circular piece of the tube about an inch in diameter—a part of two of the rings that compose the windpipe, not the whole of one—using a narrow bladed knife. Then insert a pewter, ivory, or box-wood tube, with shoulders, and holes through the shoulders, so that it may be fastened around the neck with strings. A piece of elder, three inches long, with notches cut in it, will answer the purpose.

The tube will require to be taken out from time to time and cleansed. The animal should be watched and fed on well-made gruel. In time soft food may be given, and, should the case take a favorable turn, the tube may be removed.

Should the violent effort necessary in coughing inconvenience the animal, on account of the partial escape of the air through the artificial opening, place the hand over it, and thus compel the escape of the breath through the larynx, the proper channel.

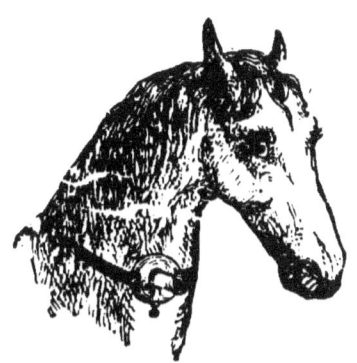

Fig. 5. The tube in use.

ERYSIPELAS

Is a specific, febrile, inflammatory disease of the skin and its subjacent tissues. Erysipelas mites (strepto-coccus erysipelatous) are said to be present. The disease is sometimes epizootic, and severe cases are frequently fatal. It is peculiar to the hind legs. The swelling is diffuse and is accompanied with eruption and great pain.

The disease differs from scarlet fever in that the swelling is uniform and firm, not in patches; from purpura in that it is local and painful, not irregularly distributed and comparatively painless; from acute farcy in that there are no corded lymphatics, and that the sores, when they exist, have no hard, circumscribed bases; from lymphangitis in that there are vesicles, sloughing sores, gangrene, and sometimes structural changes in the membrane of the mouth and upper air passages; also that it frequently begins in the region of the hock, not in the inguinal (groin) region.

Remedy.—Aperients for irritation; aconite for fever. Salines, potassium chlorate, with spirit of camphor. Hot fomentations for several hours; then moisten with borax solution and laudanum. Hypodermic injections of antiseptics sometimes limit swellings. Belladonna, internally and locally, paralyzes sensory nerves. Open all abscesses. Cleanliness, good sanitary surroundings, generous diet. Milk, eggs, beef tea, alcoholic stimulants. Ferric chloride solution, externally and locally, especially in weak patients; also quinine. (For doses, see pages 13 to 29.)

SCARLET FEVER (SCARLATINA),

Is characterized by fleabite-like scarlet spots on the mucous membrane of the nose and mouth, scattered skin eruptions—sometimes suppurations—and sore throat and neck glands. It is a sequel of other diseases—epizootic catarrh, &c. Unlike human scarlatina, it is non-contagious. There are two forms—the simple, and the complicated and severe. In the former the pulse varies from 60 to 70; in the latter 90 to 100, with great soreness of throat, a loud, moist cough, a yellowish-red mucous discharge from the nose and mouth after each cough, &c.

Remedy.—Comfortable box; light, digestible, laxative food. Water, given with sodium sulphite and hyposulphite, as antiseptics. Ammonium acetate, spirit nitrous ether and camphor in draught, thrice daily, abate fever. Medicines given in electuary when swallowing is difficult.

Inhalation of hot water vapor, medicated with antiseptics or anodynes, relieve breathing. Fomentations, woolen cloths, soaked in hot water or hot oil, for sore throat. Fomentations with hot water, mixed with sulphurous acid, for external swelling. Gargles of potassium chlorate, borax, or sulphurous acid lessen discharge and fetor from mouth and throat. Daily rubbing with vaselin or glycerine and water removes scaling crusts. Small doses of alcoholic stimulants, acid solutions of quinine or iron salts help recovery. Rest, carefully regulated, nutritive diet during convalescence. (For doses, see pages 13 to 29.)

PURPLE OR BLOOD FEVER (PURPURA HÆMORRHAGICA),

Is an eruptive, intermittent, non-contagious fever, usually, but not always, a sequel to another disease, as influenza, catarrh, or strangles. Blood issues from the flea-bite-like spots on the mucous membranes and a bloody whey from the skin swellings. The latter are painful, hot, hard, and shining, with small spots on the uncolored

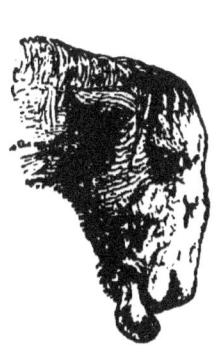
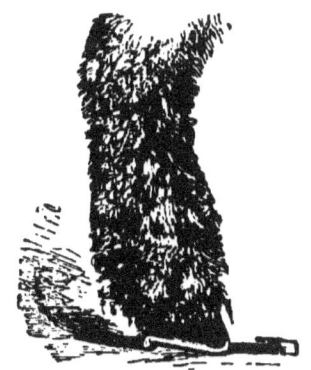

Fig. 6. Head deformed by Purple Fever (Purpura Hæmorrhagica).

Fig. 7. Leg of horse suffering from same disease.

surfaces. Vesicles about the size of a pea appear on the lower part of the limbs, and cracks at the flexures of the limbs, from which an unhealthy amber or purple colored discharge issues. The sheath, abdomen, breast, lips, nostrils, eyelids, &c., swell.

The disease is usually caused by blood contamination, but it may arise from defective drainage, ventilation, or bad food.

Remedy.—Potassium chlorate, 3 or 4 drams, 2 or 3 times daily; then half doses; usually given in drinking water. Iron salts, sulphate, perchloride; quinine, oil of turpentine. Good hygienic conditions. Concentrated, nutritive diet; oatmeal gruel, milk, eggs, alcoholic stimulants. Swellings, when limited and about head, bathed with cold water and refrigerants; when about throat, body, and legs, hot fomentations preferable, especially in cold weather. Avoid scarification unless swellings are large and causing inconvenience. Scrupulous cleanliness and antiseptic dressings while skin is ulcerating or sloughing. Open windpipe if necessary. (For doses, see pages 13 to 29.)

BRAIN AND SPINAL CORD FEVER (CEREBRO-SPINAL FEVER OR MENINGITIS),

Is a specific horse disease, characterized by congestion and inflammation of the brain and spinal cord and their nerve centers, causing paralysis, dizziness, and sudden falling to the ground. The neck and dorsal (back) muscles contract so violently as to sometimes draw the head back; the eyes are wild and injected, the head tossed about, &c. The disease is probably caused by a specific poison. It is often enzootic or epizootic, and always dangerous. In veterinary medicine 'enzootic' and 'epizootic' correspond to 'endemic' and 'epidemic' in human medicine. Enzootic diseases are local, and are confined to as well as peculiar to (if not the product of) certain districts. Epizootics are general, and may spread from country to country, like the terrible influenza epizootic of 1872-73.

Remedy.—Slings if unable to stand. Full dose of aloes; salines, laxative clyster injections, and mash diet. Small, repeated doses of alcohol and quinine for prostration. Counter-irritation to spine; ammonia and soap liniments; ice bag to spine. If urine is not passed freely, use catheter. Chloral hydrate and atrophine hypodermically relieve spasms and pain. Also ergotin and atrophine. Iron salts and strychnine for paralysis. (For doses, see pages 13 to 29.)

HORSE-POX (VARIOLA EQUINÆ),

Is a specific, contagious fever, depending on a microbe (mite) affecting the skin and mucous surfaces, and passing through papular, vesicular, and pustular stages. Rare. (Dun.) The fever is mild—continued or intermittent—and tends to self-cure.

Remedy.—Salines; antiseptics internally, cooling, laxative diet. Borax and sulphurous acid solutions abate irritation of aphthæ (roundish, pearl-colored vesicles) in mouth and throat. Lead subacetate solution, with glycerine and water, relieve skin eruptions. Isolate and disinfect. (For doses, see pages 13 to 29.)

DIPHTHERIA

Is a specific fever, characterized by inflammation of the throat, accompanied by exudation and softening of mucous surfaces. Contagious. Affects horses and dogs occasionally.

Remedy.—Ice sucked. Spray with chlorine, iodine, iodoform solutions. Ferric chloride tincture, internally and locally. Electuaries of boro-glycerine or glycerine of carbolic acid; belladonna electuaries relieve congestive stage. Sodium sulphites and hyposulphites and sulphocarbolates internally and locally. Salicylic acid and pilocarpine aid in dissolving false membrane. Soft, nutritive food; eggs, beef tea, alcohol. For doses, see pages 13 to

29. Boro-glycerine, or boro-glyceride, is made of 92 parts of glycerine to 62 of boric acid. Glycerine of carbolic acid is made of 1 part of the acid to 4 of glycerine.

A few fevers—more common to cattle than to horses—appear in Part II.

RABIES

Is a nervous, febrile disease, originating in the dog, occasionally in the cat, caused by a specific microbe (mite) in the saliva of the rabid animal. Pasteur has demonstrated that dogs and other animals inoculated with cultivated virus do not take the disease when bitten by a rabid dog, nor when inoculated with virus which would kill unprotected animals. He also claims that the cultivated virus is usually protective, if used shortly after the bite. (Dun.) Speaking of Pasteur's experiments Williams says: "If rabies be not of spontaneous origin, and if the experiments all turn out successful, there seems to be no reason why rabies should not be entirely extirpated." But he thinks the disease is sometimes spontaneous. He further says that Pasteur has succeeded "in rendering animals absolutely proof against the poison of rabies."

Symptoms.—The disease is manifested in a variety of ways. Sometimes there is great apparent distress, sudden perspirations, unruliness, stamping and pawing violently, and finally becoming frantic and dangerous. Sometimes the horse will bite the wound, tearing the skin off; intolerance of light, nervousness, eyes fixed and staring, pupils dilated; ears worked; saliva abundant. There are intervals of quiet between the fits, but they become shorter and the fits more dangerous.

Remedy.—When the disease is developed, there is no cure, but excising the wound and then cauterizing it with caustic potash or silver nitrate may possibly prevent its development.

SPASMS AND CONVULSIONS.

Spasms are involuntary muscular contractions. When attended with pain, they are called cramp. When consisting of alternate contractions and relaxations, they are called clonic spasm. When the rigidity is permanent, they are called tonic spasm, as in lock-jaw. Convulsions are muscular spasms of comparatively greater severity and extent than ordinary or local spasms, but are essentially the same in nature. The cause of the disorder is probably nervous disturbance. The fibers of a spasmed muscle feel hard and are shortened and swollen.

The disorder, which is rare, often attacks the hind legs, when it may be mistaken for spavin (concealed or not), hock disease, or patella dislocation. (The patella is the whirl-bone of the stifle joint. The whirl-bone corresponds to the knee-cap in man.) The duration of the cramp varies from minutes to hours and hours to days. Relapses are common. Sometimes the disorder is of an epileptic character (fits).

Symptoms.—When of a limb, sudden lameness; limb may be dragged, or there may be both hopping and dragging; hind leg may be caught up and thrown out in an awkward manner; standing position natural.

Remedy.—For ordinary cramp of leg, exercise. Chloral hydrate, 3 to 4 drams. Chloroform inhaled and swallowed. When of spinal origin, morphine subcutaneously (under the skin); spinal ice bag. When of cerebral (brain) origin, bromides or ammonia internally. Cold water or ice to head. When reflex, remove source of irritation. (For doses, see pages 13 to 29.)

PARALYSIS (PARESIS, PALSY),

Or loss of motor power, is a symptom of disease rather than disease itself. It is nevertheless of great importance, for it is dangerous. It is of four kinds—general, unilateral (one side), transverse (before or behind), and local. Traseverse paralysis, on account of its intimate relation to the spinal cord, is often called 'spinal paralysis.' (Robertson.)

Paralysis is caused by falls or blows, fractures or injuries, especially of the spine; overwork, blood poisoning, grass staggers, the use of the vetch known as 'lathyrus sativus,' &c. When horses are quartered in low, wet, cold pastures, especially where there is stagnant water and cold air currents, the disorder is liable to become epizootic. The attack is usually sudden. The hind legs are very susceptible to the disorder. It often affects first one leg and then the other. The sense of feeling as well as motion may be lost, which may be detected by pricks, pinches, or blows.

Symptoms—If of hind quarters, horse down, struggling with fore feet to get up; in extreme cases the rectum and bladder are also paralyzed; evacuations may be retained, but oftener pass involuntarily; when retained, remove artificially.

In complete paralysis of side, horse down on affected side; in incomplete, can stand and even drag itself along; head, neck, loins, and hind quarters incline to one side; affected eye sunken; ear lops; lips pendulous and drawn aside; drinking and mastication difficult.

In paralysis of head, the face is distorted; corners of mouth drawn upward; mastication impracticable; sight affected, but eyes retain power of motion. The disease called glass eye may follow paralysis of the head.

Remedy.—Rest, quiet. Light, digestible food. Salines, tonics. Friction, blisters, electricity, impart nervous and muscular tone. Potassium iodide and salines if dependent on pressure from fluid. Trephine and raise bone if from depression of cranial bones. Remove any gastric, uterine, or other local irritation, or blood contamination. Nux vomica and strychnine stimulate motor centers and nerves.

When caused by embolism (blood clots or foreign bodies plugging vessels), or by thrombosis (escape of a fluid and the injury caused thereby) treat the first by rest, concentrated, rather spare diet, and ammonia salts; the second by refrigerant applications or fomentations, bitters, and scarification when the swelling causes inconvenience. (For doses, see pages 13 to 29.)

TETANUS (LOCK-JAW),*

Has four forms. 1. Cramp of the muscles of the face and neck, causing the jaws to close; the most common form. 2. Cramp of the muscles of the back and loins, causing elevation of the head and sinking of the loins. 3. Bending the body and neck forward, with arching of the spine. 4. Bending the body laterally.

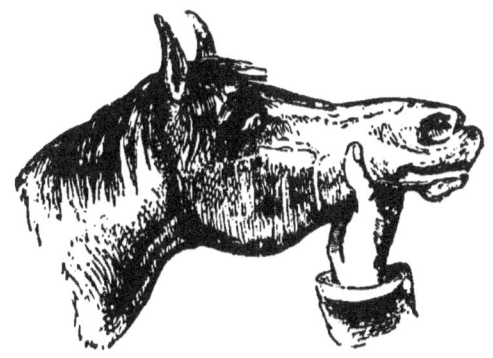

Fig. 8. Testing Tetanus. When the head is raised the haw projects over the eye.

The exact nature of the disease is still a matter of dispute. Some horses seem to be predisposed to it. The nerve centers chiefly if not solely affected are the medulla oblongata and spinal cord. The medulla oblongata lies between and connects the brain and spinal cord.

---

* Lock-jaw is only one of four different forms of Tetanus. This important fact should be borne in mind; otherwise an intelligent diagnosis (determination) of the disease is impossible.

The disease is either acute or chronic. The acute form, which usually results from wounds, is rapid in its course and very dangerous. It is perhaps sometimes spontaneous and epizootic. It attacks young as well as old, and lasts from one to three or four weeks. When curable, the turn comes in about ten days.

The disease has many causes. A nail in the foot, a mere tread, punctures, amputation of the tail, docking, saddle galls, castration, especially where caustic clamps are used; intestinal irritation, either from foreign bodies or parasites; sudden changes of temperature, especially after clipping; strychnine internally or injected; in fact, any violence. It may occur even after a wound has healed. Dun says the "involuntary tonic (rigid) muscular spasms" of tetanus are probably caused by a microbe. The mites would cause irritation of course.

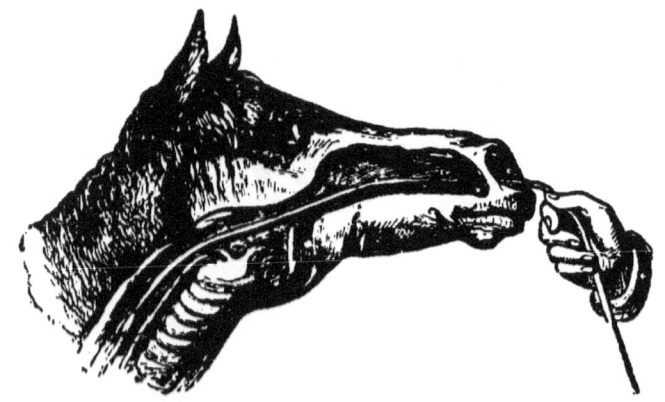

Fig. 9. Feeding a horse suffering with chronic Tetanus. A catheter passed through the nostril to the stomach; gruel pumped in.

Symptoms.—First stage: Neck, back, and loins stiff; appetite lost; swallowing difficult; lips about natural; discharge of saliva; jaws refuse to separate naturally; grinding of teeth; nose elevated and slightly protruded; facial muscles twitch; excitable, irritable; throws head up if touched; eyes watchful, brilliant, the haws, their natural shield, shooting across the eyeballs; pulse little increased, but rather hard and incompressible.

Second stage: Muscles cramped generally; head drawn upward and backward, presenting deer-like aspect; hence the name "stag-evil;" tail elevated and tremulous; limbs stretched; countenance haggard, ghastly; eyes wild, staring, protruded, haws shooting over balls, if excited; otherwise dull and sunken; ears erect, rigid; nose protruded; nostrils dilated; gait hobbling; jaws more firmly locked, &c., &c.

Third stage: Symptoms much the same, but intensified, and distress more general. Sometimes the windpipe is opened to prevent suffocation. Fatal.

Remedy.—Put in dark box; perfect quiet; loosely in slings. Aloes, aided by nutritive mashes, gruel, molasses. Salines in drinking water, kept within reach. Will suck up sloppy food even when the jaws are closed. Foment or poultice wound; remove any cause of irritation and apply anodynes. Powdered opium and cannabis indica extract, 30 grains each, softened by admixture of ammonium acetate solution, 3 times daily among molar teeth. Bromides and chloral hydrate give temporary, sometimes permanent relief. (For doses, see pages 13 to 29.)

MEGRIMS (VERTIGO, DIZZINESS, STAGGERS),

Is brain disturbance (cerebral congestion). Its usual cause is tight or badly fitting collars. This seems to be proved by the fact that horses subject to it are free of it if worked with a band across their breast; further, by the fact that loosening the collar soon stops a fit. If the collar is not loosened manually, the horse will plunge about till it falls, and thus loosen it itself. The disease has other causes, such as general plethora (too much blood) increased action of the heart, disturbed vaso-motor (vessel movement) activity, &c.

Symptoms.—Stops suddenly; shakes head either from side to side or upward and downward; head sometimes turned aside; head and throat vessels distended, their

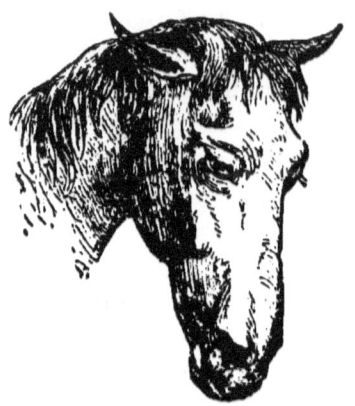

Fig. 10. Characteristic look after repeated attacks of Megrims.

respective muscles twitching rapidly; eyes stare; nostrils dilated; breathing rapid or stertorous; fore legs often wide apart, as if for support; skin damp from perspiration.

Remedy.—Treat as above stated. Cold water on head. Walking exercise. Hand-rubbing of body and legs. Moderate bleeding or physic sometimes useful.

LYMPHANGITIS OR WEED (SWELLED LEGS),

Is inflammation of the lymphatic glands, absorbent vessels and blood vessels, especially of the legs. It is peculiar, as the name indicates, to lymphatic temperaments. It is attributed to general disturbance of function, especially digestion and assimilation. Overfeeding and idleness, cold and wet, nails in the feet, inherent tendency, heredity, &c., are predisposing causes. The blood abounds in serum (a greenish yellow fluid). The second day after it is drawn the clot will swim in it. In repeated attacks the skin becomes thick and rough, as in 'elephantiasis.' Sometimes abscesses dot the limb, especially the inner part. In chronic cases the lymph glands are sometimes filled with calcareous material, grating when cut into.

The swelling of the limb is sudden, and usually reaches its hight in from 24 to 48 hours, remaining stationary equally long before declining. Any limb is susceptible to the disease, but it is a curious as well as interesting fact that the one usually affected is the left hind leg.

Symptoms.—Leg swollen, tolerably firm, hot, painful and sometimes moist, the swelling being from above downward; when severe, drops of a yellowish fluid bedew the skin; fever active, and sometimes ushered in by shivering fits; pulse 75 to 95, the artery being tense and cord-like; in severe cases the breathing is hurried, short, catching; internal temperature increased from two to five degrees; mouth clammy; bowels inclined to be confined; urine—not at first increased in quantity—is of a higher specific gravity than natural; appetite more or less impaired, with increased desire for fluids; slight restlessness, sometimes simulating colicky pains; anxious countenance; looks back repeatedly.

Remedy.—Bleed robust subjects and where fever is acute. Purge, laxative injections, and salines in drinking water. Bran mashes. Aconite for acute fever. Hot fomentations for several hours; then swathe legs lightly in woolen or hay bandages. If tender and painful, moisten with soap liniment and laudanum. Clothe well in cold weather. Stimulants where preliminary rigor is severe or continued. Exercise is injurious during acute symptoms, but serviceable later.

In hard-worked and debilitated subjects, bleeding and aconite unsuitable. Give them a half dose of physic and salines; foment leg; turpentine and alcoholic stimulants.

Aid reduction of swelling by exercise, followed by moderate work. Smart friction of leg daily, with oil. Diuretics and tonics; iodine or potassium iodide internally; laxative diet and green food.

Careful regulation of food, work, and rest diminish the chances of relapses. (For doses, see pages 13 to 29.)

HERNIA (RUPTURE),

Is a tumor or enlargement in any part of the body, caused by the protrusion, by rupture, of a viscus or part through its natural cavity. When the part can be returned to its proper cavity, the hernia is called 'reducible;' when it cannot, it is 'irreducible;' when it interferes with the circulation, it is 'strangulated.' The kind or name of the hernia depends on the part affected. The most common and important kind is

INGUINAL (GROIN) AND SCROTAL HERNIA.

It occurs in stallions, but is rare in geldings. It is comparatively rare in this country and England, but in France, Germany, India, Arabia, &c., where castration is but little practiced, it is common. The causes are overstraining of any kind, kicks, &c., but the latter is very rare. It rarely exists on both sides at once. It is peculiar to the right. Sometimes it is imperceptible, the small intestines, which are the cause of it, not protruding further than the inguinal canal. In this case feel for them. When the intestines descend to the scrotum, the hernia is called 'scrotal hernia.' Castration is necessary to a permanent cure.

When the hernia is imperceptible, the following are the

Symptoms.—Indisposition to work; head erected; appetite impaired; pain succeeding, animal breathes deeply, paws, and assumes various postures for relief. Sometimes the horse seems to be suffering from fatigue; at length pulse becomes thready; eyes reddened and pupils dilated; inflammation causes slight colic.

The symptoms of scrotal hernia are very distinct, but as the disorder is visible and the services of a surgeon are necessary, a description of them is superfluous. A case is recorded wherein the scrotum hung down nearly to the hocks.

Sometimes hernia follows castration, caused by straining perhaps. Frequently it is congenital, disappearing in from three to six months. It may exist in the fetus (fœtus.)

Remedy.—Cast, and return the bowel by hand, and if need be by application of ice or refrigerants. If this fails, enlarge constricting ring. Covered castration operation in stallion.

UMBILICAL (NAVEL) HERNIA

Is protrusion of a part of a bowel through the navel. It is peculiar to the young, and is common in breeding districts. Many require no treatment at all; others do, for they sometimes cause death. In serious cases send for a veterinary surgeon.

Remedy.—Fast for several hours; cast, place on the back, and return the protruded part. Retain in position by stitches, clamps of wood or iron, skivers or elastic ligature. Cantharides blister applied to adjacent skin causes swelling, and in slight cases shuts up opening.

VENTRAL (BELLY) HERNIA

Is caused by kicks, staking, the thrust of a horn, or other violence. It is rarely dangerous. When small and recent, the opening is usually closed by a blister. When necessary, after returning the part, cut down and stitch the opening.

Cases of artificial anus are recorded in both belly and navel hernia. Hernia of the bladder is recorded. It was as large as a man's fist, and was separated from and hung below the scrotum.

FISTULA,

A narrow, suppurating canal, may be internal or external, superficial or deep-seated, complete or incomplete, that is, have an external or internal opening only, or both. The canal may be short or a foot or more in length. Fistulæ (pleural of fistula) are caused by diseased bone, cartilage, tendon, &c., and are hard to heal.

Remedy.—Before pus is formed, reduce inflammation with cold water to the part; then iodine and a purge; do not puncture. After pus is formed, enlarge the canal with a knife; pass seton or otherwise provide dependent opening. Remove diseased bone or other irritant. Encourage healing of wound from below. Where the knife is unsuitable, inject saturated solution of corrosive sublimate, or sulphate of copper or zinc. Where milder treatment fails, slough out ulcerating surfaces and secreting walls with corrosive sublimate or arsenic plug. Dress with carbolic acid or other antiseptic. (For doses, see pages 13 to 29.)

POLL-EVIL

Is a fistulous ulcer at the poll of the neck, near the ears. From a simple swelling it develops into a tumor, from a tumor into an abscess, and from an abscess into deep-seated, chasm-like ulcers. It is caused by tight bearing-

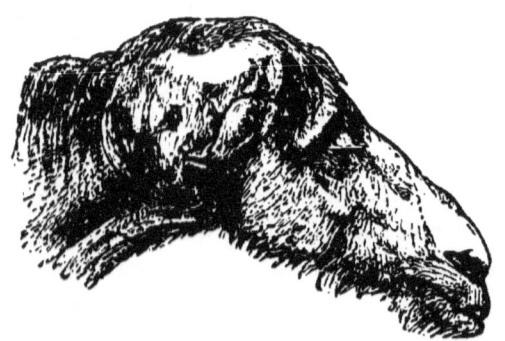

Fig. 11. Poll-Evil; ready for operation.

reins, blows, bruises, pressure, friction, &c. A stiff and hard halter or other head-gear or collar may cause friction, and a low door-way or loft floor may cause bruises. The disease is slow and hard to cure. It will penetrate to the bone, and has been known to cause pressure upon the brain.

As poll-evil is the result of mismanagement, its best remedy is the avoidance of the cause. For remedy, see 'Fistula' (page 60).

FISTULA IN THE WITHERS,

Like poll-evil, is the result of mismanagement and injuries. The withers are usually injured by saddles, harness-pads, and collars. In chronic cases, or what may be called the third stage, the disease will penetrate to and cause disease of the bone, as in poll-evil.

The first stage of the fistula is a tumor. It may be swelled, hot, and tender, or it may be indolent, manifesting neither heat nor tenderness. The former requires a cooling lotion, applied with linen; the latter, which usually has an eschar (crust or scab) on its summit, requires a bagged bran poultice, confined by a surcingle.

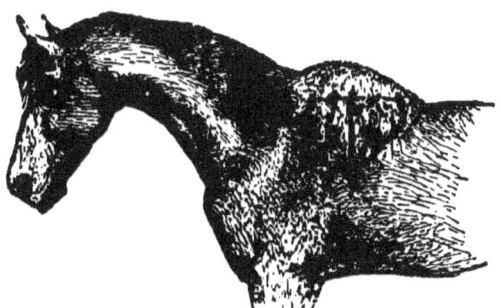

Fig. 12. Fistulous Withers; worst stage.

The formation of pus may be called the second stage of the disease. Some of the sinuses or holes are of such depth that ordinary probes are useless. When practicable, the abscess should be laid open, to afford vent for the pus. When not practicable, a counter-opening may accomplish this purpose. When practicable, setons in the fistulous canals will not only keep the apertures open, but will aid healthy granulation. Carious bone, cartilage, or ligament should be removed.

Remedy.—See 'Fistula.'

FISTULOUS PAROTID DUCT

Is rare. It is a sinuous opening, communicating with the interior of the duct, through which saliva is discharged, especially during mastication. In chronic cases the duct becomes so enlarged by the accumulation of saliva that, instead of being comparable to a goose quill, it will admit the finger. The situation of the fistula may be the angle of the bone, the inner border of the jaw, or the side of the cheek. The discharge of saliva proclaims the nature of the case. The causes of the disease are abscess of the gland, strangles (the disease), and injuries of all kinds.

Remedy.—Percivall cured two cases with the following injection: Lunar caustic, $\frac{1}{2}$ dram; nitric acid, 1 dram; distilled water, 1 ounce. Judging by experience, he recommends that the quantity of water be doubled. In the second case treated by him, the gland was destroyed. Distilled water is made as follows: Take of water 10 gallons; distill 2 pints of impurities and throw them away; then distill 8 gallons. Put in glass bottles. Distillation is the operation by which, with the aid of heat and closed vessels, the volatile or liquid parts of bodies are separated from the fixed or solid. Distillation is purification.

FISTULA OF THE ANUS,

When on account of the friction caused by the action of the muscles of the tail, is greatly benefited by confining the tail to a rope fastened around the neck, the same as horse dealers do when they link their horses together for traveling. (Percivall.)

DIABETES (POLYURIA),

Is a complex morbid condition, originating in or closely connected with certain disturbances in the process of assimilation, evidenced by excessive secretion of urine, great and persistent thirst, rapid emaciation and loss of energy, and in one form (the serious) characterized by the presence of saccharine (sugar) material in the urine. (Robertson.) Musty oats or hay, badly saved fodder, malted barley, impure water, &c., are predisposing causes. A horse has been known to drink 38 gallons of water in 5 hours. (Percivall.)

Remedy.—Half dose of physic. Iodine with potassium iodide. With iodine alternate or conjoin iron salts. Chalk or whiting in manger for acidity. Phosphoric acid and bitters lessen thirst. Change food. Moderate supply of water, with which mix sodium bicarbonate and wheaten flour or oatmeal. (For doses, see pages 13 to 29.)

RHEUMATISM

Is an inflammation of the fibrous structures of the joints, tendons, ligaments, sheaths of muscles, or of the heart and closed cavities, caused by a specific condition of the blood, and accompanied by fever, stiffness, and lameness. It is shifting or erratic in its character. (Williams) It is believed to depend on the accumulation in the body of some product of nutritive derangement, probably lactic (milk) acid. (Dun.) Cold, dampness, predisposition, the debility caused by other diseases, and heredity are its chief causes perhaps.

Remedy.—Alkalies, potassium bicarbonate and nitrate in drinking water. Ammonium acetate and colchicum. Hot fomentations or flannels wrung out of hot water or oil to affected parts. Then moisten with aconite, opium, or other anodynes. When acute symptoms abate, quinine, arsenic, Donovan's solution internally. Quiet, comfortable quarters. Flannels soaked with hot oil and alkaline solutions, kept on for 1 or 2 hours, for stiffness and swelling. Then soap liniment. Light work. If mild remedies fail, apply cantharides ointment. Actual cautery sometimes required in chronic articular (joint) rheumatism. No bleeding. (For doses, see pages 13 to 29.) Actual cautery means the application of a red hot iron.

BARRENNESS.

Remedy.—Change diet and surroundings. Exercise. Alteratives; potassium iodide; phosphorus and cantharides, small doses. Gradual reducing of fat, plethoric subjects. Good diet and tonics for debilitated. Dilate os uteri if it be impervious. Change male. (For doses, see pages 13 to 29.) The 'os uteri' is the mouth of the womb.

DROPSIES,

Says Percivall, may arise from general or local plethora, obstructed circulation, deficient absorption, or a thin or watery condition of the blood. They are either external or internal, acute or chronic. External dropsy is a collection of watery fluid in the cellular membrane beneath the skin. In internal dropsy the fluid fills the cavities of the body—the chest, belly, head, &c.

Dropsy is the result of vascular (vessel) disturbance. Vascular disturbance is therefore the exciting cause of dropsy; debility is the predisposing cause.

"Turned out" horses are often dropsical. They exchange a warm atmosphere for a cold and moist one, a generous for a low diet, and sometimes wholesome for unwholesome water.

DROPSY OF THE ABDOMEN OR PERITONEUM (ASCITES),

The peritoneum is a watery membrane lining the abdominal cavity. Anything that disturbs its healthy action, such as disease of the liver, heart, kidneys, spleen, or omentum (a prolongation of the peritoneum); improper or insufficient food, exposure to cold, &c., may cause dropsy. It is sometimes complicated with hydrothorax and dropsy of the pericardium—a sequel sometimes of the latter. The pale, straw-colored fluid—aggregating gallons—is sometimes mixed with flakes of lymph. The disease is peculiar to the young rather than the old.

Symptoms.—Dull; if in the field, alone; appetite and general condition bad; disposed to rest; abdomen becomes gradually pendulous; pulse weak and rather frequent; membranes blanched. These symptoms may become intensified and multiplied, the swelling extending to the limbs, &c. When the liver is much diseased, the urine is always scanty and biliary; when the kidneys are diseased, it is charged with albumen.

Remedy.—Diuretics, salines, oil of turpentine. Digitalis in heart complications. Combat liver complications. (See liver diseases.) Tapping gives relief.

Shelter, good food, some exercise. Cautious use of preparations of iron. When bowels confined, moderate doses of aloes at long intervals, or sulphate of soda steadily. For albumen in urine, perchloride or sulphate of iron, with dilute sulphuric acid, alternated with solution of iodine or iodide of potassium—one in morning, other at night—using diuretics, if at all, sparingly. Remove local swelling by fomentation, smart friction, with simple oil, and moderate exercise. For chronic, debilitated cases, 2, 3, or even 4 ounces cod-liver oil, twice a day, mixed with 4 or 5 eggs. (For doses, see pages 13 to 29.)

DROPSIES, GENERAL (ANASARCA),

Swell the legs, sheath, breast, belly, lips, eyelids, &c. They are often the result of either constitutional disease or deficiency and poverty of blood. They are external—beneath the skin—but in chronic cases there may be internal accumulations also, and sometimes sympathetic inflammation of the air passages. The latter is a very dangerous complication. The swellings have a soft feel and pit on pressure. Dullness, loss of appetite, strength, and flesh, short and difficult breathing, and frequent and indistinct pulse are characteristic symptoms.

Remedy.—Turkish baths. Digitalis infusion and strychnine are useful in most dropsies, especially in dropsy of the heart, in which give with salines. Copaiba in heart and liver cases. Laxatives and potassium iodide in kidney cases. Encourage vicarious functions of bowels and skin in kidney cases. Iron and salines for lack of blood. Friction, shampooing, external stimulants. Draw off water with trocar. Also with aspirator (injection-like syringe). Acupuncture (the introduction of needles into the living tissues for remedial purposes.)

For doses, see pages 13 to 29.

DROPSY OF THE SCROTUM (HYDROCELE),

Is rare.

Remedy.—Evacuate by trocar and canula. Injection of iodine or other astringent solution.

SEROUS ABSCESS

Is a kind of dropsy. It is usually situated on the outer side of the thigh, in front of the stifle, the breast, the shoulder, and the arm. Though circumscribed, the abscesses are occasionally of considerable size. Their shape is ovoid, flattened upon the surface. They have a soft, fluctuating feel, and, when punctured, emit a jet of straw-colored fluid, very like the serum (water or whey) of the blood. They are caused by blows or other contusions. Percivall suggests that there may be another kind of serous abscess—one that arises spontaneously.

Remedy.—Do not attempt to disperse these tumors. Lance them. Inject with one of the following mixtures: 1. White vitriol, 1 scruple; distilled water, 1 ounce. 2. Lunar caustic, 1 scruple; distilled water, 1 ounce. Or pass a seton through the enlargement. After the injection, or after the withdrawal of the seton, a compress and roller will agglutinate the sides of the cavity. The seton should be retained only till healthy pus is produced. In some cases, especially where a bandage cannot be kept on nor a seton be inserted, sloughing the sac with a sharp escharotic (caustic), such as powdered blue vitriol, is the best means of cure. (Percivall.)

GLANDERS AND FARCY

Is a malignant, contagious, and fatal disease, due to the introduction into the animal economy, or of generation within it, of a virus (said by Dr. Struck of Berlin to consist of an organism, the 'Bacillus mallei,' about the same size as those of tuberculosis), which, infecting the whole system, shows specific effects on the nasal membrane, the lungs, and the lymphatic glands and ducts. It originates spontaneously in the horse, ass, and mule, and is transmissible to sheep, goats, dogs, cats, mice, and rabbits; also to man, in whom the virus seems to increase in malignancy. Cattle, swine, and fowl resist it, even when inoculated. It may occur under at least four forms—acute and chronic glanders; acute (bud) and chronic (button) farcy. (Williams.)

Old age, bad food and management, overwork, exhausting diseases, such as diabetes insipidus; specific miasmatic or animal poisons, especially those of overcrowded stables, &c., are believed to be predisposing causes of glanders.

The discharge from the nostrils caused by caries of the nasal bones and the roots of the upper molar teeth (the back molars), is sometimes mistaken for glanders. This need not be if the following facts are noted: In glanders the discharge, *at first*, is never fetid; in caries it is always fetid. In glanders, however, the discharge becomes very offensive in the course of time. The latter fact is very valuable in a diagnostic point of view.

When described as distinct diseases, glanders is said to affect the nasal membrane, farcy the skin.

Remedy.—Dress farcy buds with mercuric iodide ointment or stick of silver nitrate. Sodium hyposulphite; iron and copper sulphates; arsenic internally. Liberal diet; exercise desirable, except in acute cases. Isolate from healthy animals; disinfect. Treatment only palliative. Better slaughter. (For doses, see pages 13 to 29.)

OSTEOPOROSIS (HARDENING),

Consists in the excessive development of the tissues which occupy the canals and cells of bones, while at the same time the actual quantity of bony matter remains unaltered. (Rokitansky.) From perverted nutrition the bones are thus swollen and brittle. The cartilaginous tissues, and even the teeth, undergo similar degeneration. The disease occurs in horses, cattle, and sheep.

Incurable. Prevention consists in furnishing food containing a proper proportion of all the elements of nutrition.

FLYBLOW (Magots from),

If neglected, may result in death. Sheep suffer more perhaps than horses.

Remedy.—Turpentine; tar oil; corrosive sublimate solution.

RICKETS (RACHITIS),

Is faulty development and softening (causing bending) of the bones of young animals, depending on disordered nutrition of the osseous (bony) tissue; in fact, to the mal-assimilation and non-development of the materials necessary to the formation of bone—namely, phosphate and carbonate of lime.

Rickets appears when the patient is a few weeks or months old, and is caused by constitutional debility, scrofulous taint, or by external and preventable causes. Thus we find it in calves that are not allowed to suckle their mother, and in foals that suckle but two or three times a day, the mother being at work. Young animals fed on artificial food instead of milk, and not allowed proper exercise, or reared under any unnatural conditions, are liable to become rickety.

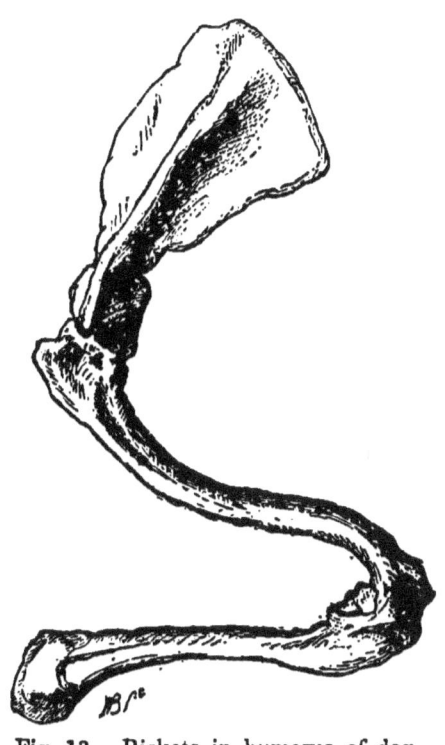

Fig. 13. Rickets in humerus of dog.

Remedy.—Nourishing diet. Milk, crushed oats, with linseed, for horses, cattle, sheep, swine. Milk, meat soup, cod-liver oil for dogs. In sucking animals, see to quality and quantity of milk. An aperient or antacids will rectify digestive derangement. Calcium phosphate; Parrish's food; iron salts; healthy surroundings. Splints and bandages if needed. (For doses, see pages 13 to 29.)

DISEASES OF THE AIR PASSAGES.

The air passages are the nostrils, the larynx, the windpipe and its ramifications, and the bronchial tubes. The horse, on account of the great size of the soft palate, cannot breathe through its mouth. The chambers of the nose are therefore exposed to noxious effluvias in the air, while the mouth is exempt. This difference from man in structure and economy probably accounts for the proneness of the horse to pulmonary affections. The nasal membrane should be frequently inspected. In health it displays a dotted, shining, humid aspect, of a more or less flesh color. Mucus is a sign of disease.

CATARRH,

An unhealthy discharge from the nose, in the membrane of which it has its seat, is usually if not invariably the result of cold—that is, cold that causes unusual suffering. Percivall says that catarrh is much oftener the result of transition from cold to heat than from heat to cold; also that horses kept in the open air altogether are hardly susceptible to catarrh.

The disease is peculiar to young horses and is sometimes epizootic. It is common, but it is usually harmless. However, it should not be neglected, for it may lead to bronchitis, nasal gleet, roaring, &c.

Simple and Febrile Symptoms.—Sneezing; redness and dryness of nasal membrane; watery, irritating discharge, becoming in a few days turbid, yellowish, and irregular; redness of conjunctival (eye) membrane; copious tears; hanging head; yawning; heat and pain over frontal sinuses; small, loose, diffuse swellings under jaw; sometimes coughing, with or without soreness of throat; varying degrees of fever, dullness, and debility; staring coat; rigors or shivering fits; surface temperature now elevated, now depressed; internal temperature elevated 3 or 4 degrees; pulse and breathing quickened; appetite diminished. As the acute symptoms subside, the disease becoming subacute or established as it were, the animal improves. In some cases the symptoms are much more severe than above described, sometimes threatening suffocation.

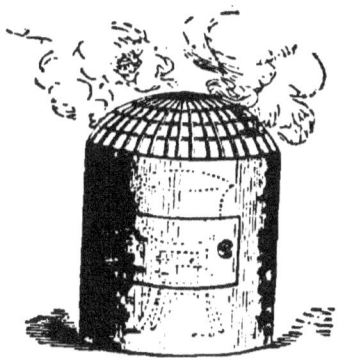

Fig. 14. Steaming apparatus for Catarrh, Bronchitis, &c.

Chronic Symptoms.—The discharge is considerably altered in character, and is for a time at least less in quantity; but the quantity varies—more one day than another. Sometimes the discharge is white and glairy; sometimes a yellow mixture of pus and mucus; in rare cases, opaque, thin, dirty-looking mucus; appetite good, but animal lacks bloom, vigor, vivacity; coat open; skin scurfy; nasal membrane rather soft, blanched, thickened, and less vascular-looking, and of a slate or leaden hue.

Remedy.—Simple form: House comfortably; clothe body and head; bandage legs. Temperature 60 to 65° F. Steam head with vapor of water alone, or medicated with antiseptic or anodyne. Warm or vapor bath; dry quickly and reclothe; mash diet or green food; laxative injections; purge if necessary. Ammonia acetate solution; potassium nitrate and chlorate; other saline electuaries. Hot fomentations; stimulating embrocations to throat.

Chronic form: Isolate; rest or light work; if the coat is rough, clip or singe. Arsenic, iron, copaiba, terrebene improve general condition. Inhalation or spray of sulphurous or carbolic acid or iodoform. Astringent nasal douche or spray; blister over nasal sinuses. (For doses, see pages 13 to 29.)

SORE THROAT (LARYNGITIS),

Is a rather common, rapid, and dangerous disease. The inflammation usually extends to the pharynx and contiguous parts. The swelling and mucous accumulations sometimes cause death by suffocation. The causes are the same as those of catarrh and bronchitis, and most of the effects and complications are the same also. Long-continued and hacking coughs are frequently present.

Robertson divides the disease into two forms—catarrhal and swollen. He also speaks of a chronic form, consisting of muscular wasting and degeneration, with adventitious growth and changes of inherent tissue—the same as in roaring.

Symptoms.—Head elevated and protruded; more or less difficulty in swallowing; ropy and tenacious saliva; cough at first hard and rather sonorous; as the disease advances and the secretion increases, it is less resonant, rather suppressed, and emitted with evidence of pain. More or less fever; restless; stamps, tosses head, pulls backward. Pulse high, eyes prominent, legs and ears cold. Spasms of the larynx sometimes occur, followed by great difficulty in breathing, loud, shrill, trumpet-like sounds, &c.

Purple-hued nasal membrane, difficulty in breathing, stupor, anxiety, restlessness, &c., according to Robertson, are characteristic of the swollen form of laryngitis.

Remedy.—Comfortable box and clothing; protect from drafts; moist atmosphere of 60 to 70° F. Steam head and throat persistently with medicated vapor; heat and moisture externally. Aconite and laxatives abate fever in early stages of acute attacks. Emetics relieve fever and difficult breathing in dogs and pigs. Ammonium acetate solution, camphor, and belladonna confections. Benzoin, sulphurous acid, iodine, or chloroform as inhalation, spray, or confection. Salicylic acid and potassium chlorate as confection every hour where swelling is great. Counter-irritants—soap and opium liniment, mustard, cantharides. Tube in windpipe if necessary.

Chronic form: Alum, ferric chloride, sulpho-carbolates, or tannic acid as confection or spray. Belladonna and camphor, with glycerine and water, as anodyne gargle. Thickening of mucous membrane treated by potassium iodide and counter-irritants. Essence of mustard hypodermically. Ulceration of the opening of the glottis (rima glottidis) treated with silver nitrate.

For doses, see pages 13 to 29.

NASAL GLEET (OZENA OR OZŒNA),

Is usually preceded by an inflammatory or catarrhal attack, but it may occur spontaneously. It is more likely to follow chronic than acute catarrh. It is peculiar to adult or old horses rather than young. It is sometimes mistaken for glanders.

In most cases the discharge, which is usually from both nostrils, continues long after inflammation has ceased. It is more mucous than purulent, is remarkably white, and about as thick as cream. Sometimes it is smooth and uniform; sometimes lumpy; at others it is yellow, and seems to contain more pus than mucus. Sometimes it will collect about the nostrils and be ejected, in pretty regular succession, in flakes or masses. Again it is irregular, ceasing for a while, as if cured, then returning in double or treble the quantity. Sometimes the lower jaw glands are swollen, sometimes not. Sometimes there is an offensive smell, sometimes not. The nasal membrane becomes pallid and leaden-hued, but is free from pus or ulcers. Health, spirits, and appetite good. (Percivall.)

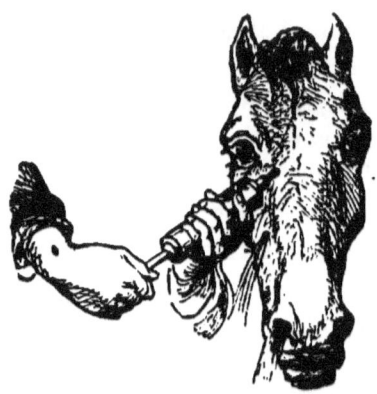

Fig. 15. Injecting for Nasal Gleet. Holes made by trephine.

Remedy.—Sulphurous acid, iodine, iodoform inhalations. Nasal douches of salt and water, with a few drops of iodine tincture. Bleaching powder scattered in box. Copper or iron sulphates, arsenic, turpentine, buchu, copaiba internally. Blister over sinuses. Remove bad teeth. When other treatment fails, trephine sinuses; after removing as much pus as possible, wash out with antiseptics. Isolate all horses with suspicious nasal discharges.

For doses, see pages 13 to 29.

ROARING

Is a symptom of disease rather than disease. It is a species of unsoundness, and may be detected sometimes by a mere fright—sudden jump; sometimes great exertion is needed. Veterinarians detect it sometimes by a grunting or groaning cough, which they produce by grasping the throat. It is sometimes hereditary. "The produce of certain sires are nearly all roarers." (Williams.) It may depend on thickening of the mucous lining of the nares (apertures), pharynx, or larynx, or on fibrous growths in these regions; but the majority of cases are the result of paralysis, wasting, and fatty degeneration of the whole of the intrinsic muscles of the left side of the larynx supplied by the recurrent nerve. The tube through which the air passes being narrowed, the characteristic noise is produced. Most roarers are wheezers, and also grunters, and in the lighter breeds are whistlers. (Dun.)

Percivall ligatured a horse's windpipe moderately tight. It roared when trotted. He next compressed the pipe to about half its natural calaber. The animal whistled. He then drew the cord with all his strength. A minute afterward the horse staggered a good deal, fell, struggled violently, and expired in two minutes after falling. The ligatured part of the windpipe admitted a crow's quill. In the two first experiments the sounds were louder in inspiration than expiration.

Remedy.—'Spurious roaring,' depending on cold, influenza, or strangles, is sometimes treated successfully by stimulation of the throat, and by potassium iodide and arsenic internally.

'True roaring,' depending on muscular wasting, is incurable. Smart blistering, the actual cautery, and galvanism in the earlier stages, sometimes retard wasting. Slow, easy work. A pad fitted on the nostrils, regulating the supply of air, lessens the noise. A tube in the windpipe affords relief. (See Fig. 5.) Removal of the paralyzed vocal cord is useless. Removal of the aretenoid cartilage is seldom permanently effectual.

For doses, see pages 13 to 29.

COUGH

Is symptomatic of various diseases. It may remain after its cause is removed. It sometimes becomes chronic, especially if neglected.

Remedy.—Comfortable housing and clothing, pure air, careful feeding, oleaginous diet.

Catarrhal: Steam head; ammonium acetate solution, salines, ether, mustard to throat.

Bronchial: Ammonium acetate, ipecac, squill, nitrous ether, counter-irritants.

Dry, with scanty secretion: Ammonium acetate or chloride, potassium bicarbonate and chlorate, borax.

With profuse discharges: Balsams, eucalyptus oil, tar, terrebene, creosote, astringent sprays or inhalations.

Irritable: Demulcents; camphor and belladonna, conium, opium, hydrocyanic acid, cocaine. (For a list of demulcents, see page 33.)

Reflex: Bromides, chloral hydrate. Remove cause of irritation.

Chronic: Careful dieting; wet the food; linseed mash or oil. If the coat is long, clip or singe. Epsom salt or other salines occasionally. Dick's recipe—30 grains each of calomel, digitalis, opium and camphor. Omit calomel if given daily for a week, that is, if necessary. Belladonna, camphor, alcohol, tar, creosote, arsenic. Counter-irritants—mustard, mercuric iodide ointment, setons.

For doses, see pages 13 to 29.

BLEEDING FROM THE NOSE (EPISTAXIS),

Is best distinguished perhaps from bleeding of the lungs by the fact that blood usually issues from but one nostril. Blood may flow in a stream or drop by drop. In either case it is very apt to collect within the chambers of the nose and about the nostril and cause irritation. The horse will snort and blow out clots of blood, and thus increase the bleeding. The blood is mostly arterial —usually a bright scarlet.

The cause may be constitutional, local, spontaneous— the result of plethora or congestion—or traumatic (wounds).

D'Arboval reports fatal cases, wherein the clots of blood in the chambers of the nose resembled pus.

Remedy.—When from rupture of small blood vessel, plug nostril and raise head. Ice to face and head. Ferric chloride tincture in spray. When from purpura or a similar disease, ergot, ferric chloride, or pyrogallic acid internally, or ergotin under the skin.

For doses, see pages 13 to 29.

NASAL POLYPUS

Is very rare in horses. "Manifold are the dangers of the distemper," says Vegetius (about 400 A. D.) "The horse will be strangled by the stoppage of the passage of his breath. He will snore, and humid mucus will flow out of his nostrils." Percivall says the mucus is sometimes highly tinged with blood, and that sometimes pure blood runs from the nose. Also that an unequal rush of air is felt from one or both nostrils. "Inspection in a full light discloses, higher or lower in the nostril, the rounded base of a polypus." He warns veterinarians not to mistake the cartilaginous prolongation of either the anterior or posterior turbinated bones for a polypus; nor any rounded clots of blood near them.

The tumors, which vary in weight from a few drams to three or four pounds, hang by a narrow neck. Sometimes they protrude three or four inches. They are red or flesh-like in color, globular in shape, and have smooth, shining surfaces. Some have a fibrous, almost cartilaginous, structure, while "others appear to be composed of various little tumors agglutinated together."

Remedy.—Excise with forceps. Dress antiseptically. Pads over nostrils sometimes diminish noise. (For a list of antiseptic remedies, see page 31.)

BRONCHOCELE OR GOITER (Tumor of the Thyroid Gland),

Is rare in horses. It is usually small and harmless, but when it increases to the size of a hen's egg or larger, it may cause choking. Percivall reduced such a swelling by rubbing with compound iodine ointment daily for six weeks, but he was in doubt whether the tumor caused the choking or not.

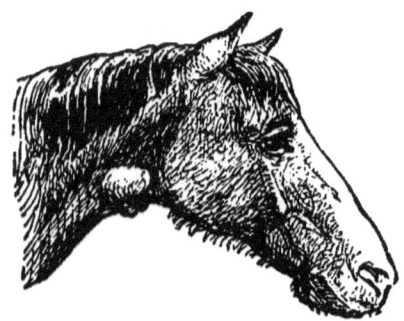

Fig. 16. Bronchocele.

The tumor, as the illustration shows, appears just below the part grasped to excite coughing. It is circular or ovoid in shape, and is soft, puffy, moveable, and devoid of sensibility.

DISEASES OF THE LUNGS.

THE lungs, though very susceptible to disease, possess comparatively little sensibility, either in health or disease. They are peculiar to themselves, and are extremely varied in structure. The bronchial tubes constitute one part; the air-cells, in which the tubes terminate, another; their blood vessels a third; the inter-connecting parenchymatous substance a fourth; the cellular and pleural membranes a fifth. In health they possess a pale pink, spongy, light, and elastic interior, and will float in water. In disease they are reddened and solidified (liver-like), and sink in water.

In horses diseases of the lungs are more numerous in proportion to other diseases than in man. They are also more rapid in their course, death sometimes resulting in a few hours. Young horses are more subject to them than old. High-bred, tenderly reared, light bodied, long legged, flat sided, narrow breasted, and thin skinned horses are more predisposed to them than those of the opposite kind. The causes of them are chiefly foul air, especially when combined with heat; sudden changes of temperature, dampness, overwork, and mechanical and chemical injuries. (Percivall.)

PNEUMONIA

Means either congestion or inflammation of the lungs, independent or combined. Inflammatory pneumonia is either simple or compound. When complicated with bronchitis, it is called 'broncho-pneumonia;' when complicated with pleurisy, 'pleuro-pneumonia.' Its progress will vary according to circumstances. Usually it reaches its hight in a few days, and gets better or worse in a few days. (Percivall.)

Robertson and Williams describe congestion as a distinct and sometimes independent disease.

Symptoms of Congestive Pneumonia.—Sudden or gradual. When sudden—the result of overexertion—the horse is all over in a tremor; cold sweat; no pulse; legs deathly cold; the frightfully wild look of the eyes—pupils dilated—and the boring of the head and stupidity of the horse, clearly indicate delirium. When gradual, the horse is at first dull, listless, heavy-headed, and off its appetite. Respiration gradually becomes more disturbed and oppressive, partaking more of labor than of pain; pulse full and quick, but so feeble perhaps as to be hardly perceptible; respiratory murmur lost; legs and ears deathly cold; cold sweats; gradually sinks, and dies in convulsions and delirium.

Remedy.—Immediate bleeding—4 to 6 quarts.

Symptoms of Inflammatory Pneumonia.—There are three stages; the first may be either absent or unnoticed. First stage: Staring coat; legs cold, followed perhaps by rigor; head hangs; no appetite; has had a short, dry cough for several days, which comes on after exercise or drinking; dull, dejected, laggard. Temperature 103, 104, or even 106. Now come fever, quick pulse, hot mouth, injected membranes of nose and eyes.

Second stage: Breathing disturbed; nostrils open and shut; flanks work laboriously up and down; breathing indicates oppression rather than pain or rapidity. In other cases the flanks hardly move at all. The nostrils are an important guide, as there is often a sparing, yellow, slimy discharge from one or both; pulse, at first, quick and usually distinct, but, as the disease progresses, is very apt, from fullness and oppression, to become indistinct; ears and legs colder than ever; nasal membrane moist and reddened; horse sometimes stands constantly in the same place and posture, fore legs stretched out, head toward a door or open window, looking backward from time to time at its heaving flanks in a peculiarly despondent manner; never lies down.

Third stage: Respiration quicker and more oppressed; pulse quicker, but less distinct; extremities cold; nasal

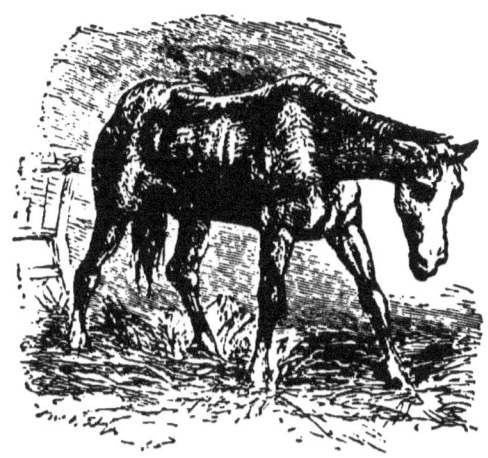

Fig. 17. Usual position during a serious attack of Pneumonia.

membrane changes from red to a leaden hue; convulsive twitchings of the muscles of the surface; extreme uneasiness; up and down; reeling gait; haggard countenance; delirium, convulsions, death.

Auscultation, according to D'Arboval, reveals a crepitating, humid rattle around the inflamed places, with a louder respiratory murmur than in other parts. Percussion reveals deadness in diseased parts, resonance in others. When the roots only of the lungs are inflamed, these tests are not present. Robertson says the heart sounds are also intensified over the consolidated (lung) area.

Remedy.—Box; temperature 60 to 70° F. Clothe body, bandage legs. Cold linseed tea; steamed food; fresh grass for horses, cattle, sheep. Bleeding in acute attacks if patient is robust. A few small doses of aconite tincture for acute fever. If fever of low type, as it usually is in hard worked town horses, sulphuric or nitric ethers, with camphor and ammonium carbonate, in draft; while ammonium acetate, potassium chlorate and nitrate are given in draft or drinking water. Potassium nitrate and colchicum for kidneys when not acting. Rugs wrung out of hot water to sides, with subsequent rubefacient dressing. Alcoholic stimulants, ether, nitrous ether, spirit of chloroform several times daily when melting of exudate (oozing matter) has begun, or earlier in epizootic attacks, or in weakly patients. Belladonna extract and camphor allay cough. Linseed oil in mash, neutral salts in drinking water, with laxative injections, secure regularity of bowels. If laxatives necessary, oil preferable to aloes. Cooling mash diet in earlier stages; in later, digestible, nutritive food. For doses, see pages 13 to 29. For list of 'rubefacients,' see page 36.

CHRONIC PNEUMONIA

May be a continuation of the acute form. It is insidious in its symptoms and dangerous; but it is mild, and its progress is slow. It may end in solidification or induration, or in tubercles, abscesses, and consumption, the same as the acute form described above.

Symptoms.—Horse appears to be merely unwell; no perceptible heaving of flanks; but little acceleration of pulse; no apparent pain, yet mopes about, dull and dejected; appetite fastidious; seldom or never lies down; coat unkind; general appearance unhealthy. Ask about cough. Examine nostrils for disturbed respiration, and also for expectoration from them.

BRONCHITIS

Means inflammation of the bronchial tubes—the two lung branches of the windpipe. It is dangerous only when

BRONCHITIS.

its secretions clog the tubes, choking the horse to death, or when it is complicated with other diseases. The latter is unfortunately frequently the case, for it is often complicated with catarrh, sore throat, and diseases of the lungs. In fact, the causes of catarrh are the causes of bronchitis. Bronchitis is simply catarrh of the bronchial tubes.

The disease rarely exists independently. It is acute, subacute, and sometimes chronic. In the spring and fall it is sometimes epizootic, especially among young horses. When acute and favorable, it reaches its hight about the fourth or fifth day; begins to decline about the sixth or seventh day, leaving the patient out of danger about the tenth or twelfth. If not favorable, the signs on the fifth, seventh, or ninth day are: Respiration becoming very oppressed; pulse quicker and fainter; skin and extremities cold; mouth cold and clammy; nostrils very dry. Pulmonic or pleuro-pulmonic disease may now supervene.

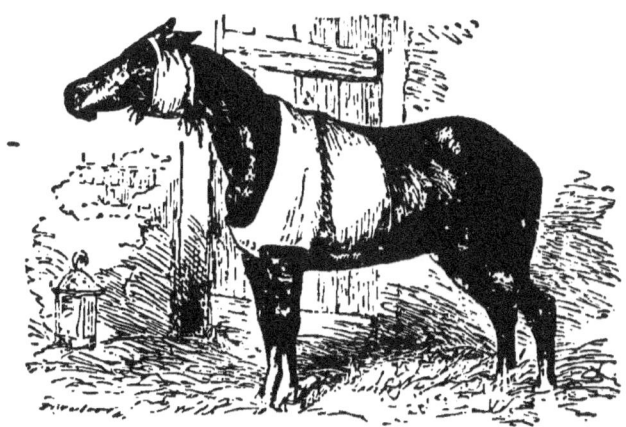

Fig. 18. A horse dressed for Bronchitis.

Symptoms.—Breath hot; unusual nasal discharge; reddening of nasal membrane; cough; sore throat; difficult breathing; febrile irritation, sometimes without antecedent shivering. Auscultation reveals a distinct cooing sort of sound, arising from want of secretion within the tubes. When the secretion returns, and in augmented quantity, the rattle is distinctly heard.

In catarrhal bronchitis, in addition to most of the above symptoms, the nasal discharge, which at first is but slight and of a watery or muco-watery description, in three or four days becomes of a puro-mucous nature and increased in quantity. The symptoms of catarrh and sore throat gradually abate and merge into that short and laborious breathing which clearly denotes high bronchial and pulmonary irritation. When the horse coughs, which it does more now, an increased discharge is expelled from the nose; when it hangs its head, the discharge runs out.

Symptoms of independent (uncomplicated) bronchitis: Sudden illness; violent blowing and distressful breathing; sudden and copious mucous discharges from the nose; may obtain relief at the moment, but there is danger of suffocation, especially if the discharges are frequently repeated. These sudden and violent attacks usually soften down to ordinary bronchitis, but they sometimes increase in violence and end in pulmonary disease.

Epizootic symptoms: Exceedingly sore throat and profuse discharges from nose; sometimes white, sometimes yellow, sometimes even green, according to circumstances. The green tinge arises either from malignancy or green food. Great weakness of loins; also general weakness; low febrile irritation.

Remedy.—Comfortable, cool, well ventilated box; temperature 60 to 65° F. Body and limbs clothed. Inhalation of watery vapor from steam kettle, a large mash, or bucket of boiling water promotes exudation in dry stage, the inhalation to be medicated, as required, with expectorants, anodynes, or antiseptics. (See Fig. 14.) Fomentations and mustard to throat and sides. Mustard in earlier stages applied for 15 or 20 minutes, washed off, and reapplied if needed. Spirituous essence of mustard injected hypodermically. Salines in drinking water for fever. A few doses of aconite early in robust subjects, where the symptoms are acute. Ammonium acetate solution, ipecac, and squill while membrane is dry and congested. Benzoic acid, eucalyptus oil, terebene, pilocarpine, mineral acids diminish excessive secretion. Soap liniment and laudanum rubbed into throat and down neck twice daily for difficult breathing, especially when the secretion is excessive. Belladonna stimulates respiratory center and eases cough; often conjoined with camphor, ether, chloral hydrate, and in debilitated patients with small, repeated doses of alcohol. Confections or gargles of opium, chloral hydrate, with glycerine, for cough. Potassium chlorate and ammonium chloride promote fluid secretion and moderate its quantity. Lobelia and opium where there is much discharge and paroxysms of cough. Ammonium carbonate when mucus is abundant and viscid and patient is low. Mash diet. Regulate bowels, if possible, by injections; purgatives dangerous in horses.

Remedy for Chronic Bronchitis.—Equable temperature; pure, fresh air; comfortable clothing, which must be removed and patient wisped over night and morning. Salines, with or without mercurials, for congestion and fever. Terebene and eucalyptus oil stimulate bronchial secretion. Belladonna, balsams, and mineral acids diminish excessive secretion. Ammonium carbonate and chloride for viscid and irritating secretion. Belladonna and ether stimulate respiratory and heart centers. Chloroform, chloral, and opium abate cough. Mustard and other counter-irritants, carefully used, lessen congestion, irritation, and cough. Mustard in-rubbing. Soap liniment, with or without laudanum, often removes cough. Alcohol, ether, volatile oils, digitalis maintain heart action in weakly subjects. Sulphurous acid, creosote, eucalyptus, and other antiseptics inhaled or internally when secretions are fetid. Arsenic occasionally relieves inflation. Careful dietary; nutritive, oleaginous food. Linseed oil. Iron and other tonics promote convalescence.

For doses, see pages 13 to 29.

PLEURISY (PLEURITIS),

Is inflammation of the pleura—a membrane investing the organs of the chest. When the inflammation extends to the lungs, the disease is called pleuro-pneumonia. The secretions of the pleura are usually watery, with or without lymph. The water is usually of a clear, bright yellow color, closely resembling the serum of the blood, though in some cases it is rendered turbid by the lymph floating in it. In others it is red from being tinged with blood. In others still it is of a sort of milky or whey color, and fetid from being mixed with pus. The lymph consists of masses of gelatinous or albuminous matter, hanging about the chest in shreds "after the fashion of a cobweb," and sometimes forming what are called adhesions or false membranes. It sometimes walls the water in as it were, confining it like pus within an abscess. It at first probably gives rise to more or less pain, as it interferes with the free action of the lungs, but the parts evidently soon become adjusted to each other. Pus sometimes accompanies acute as well chronic pleurisy, and in some cases gangrene and even abscess of the side supervene. In chronic cases the pleura becomes thickened and tough, apparently less vascular, and assumes a morbidly white aspect. Sometimes it is studded with tubercle-like knots. Pleurisy of one side is rare; but the opposite side often takes the disease from sympathy.

The disease has a dangerous tendency. It usually comes and goes suddenly. Death is also sudden—a few hours. The chronic form is slow and comparatively painless. It may last for weeks. It may follow or be independent of the acute form. The disease is peculiar to four and five-year-old horses, especially such as are kept in warm stables and live high.

The causes are cold, immersion of legs in or drinking cold water when heated, sympathy with contiguous inflammatory diseases, blood contamination, morbid growths, external injury to membrane, overexertion, &c.

Williams describes 'epizootic pleurisy,' which is "preceded and accompanied by a low typhoid or adynamic (sinking) form of fever." It lasts from one to two weeks.

Symptoms.—Slight chill or rigor; fever; uneasiness, gradually increasing till acute pain is manifested, when the animal heaves or rather pants violently at the flanks, puffs, blows, and casts piteous looks at its flanks; heat all over body, in parts actually sweating with pain; great nervous irritation; cannot be quiet for a minute; looks here and there, pawing, lying down, getting up. Pressure on the rib spaces causes flinching, usually a characteristic grunt, and an attempt to bite; a cough is often present, causing such pain that the animal, in its effort to suppress it, makes a sort of reiterated, hacking, half-cough of it; pulse very quick, firm, and wiry; mouth hot and dry; breath cold; nasal membrane reddened and moist; no discharge, unless some catarrhal or bronchial irritation be also present.

When there is inflammation of the muscles (pleurodynia) the horse moves in a very rigid manner; may fall; steps slowly and very short; dejected; back arched; skin tender.

In the chronic form the symptoms are mostly very different, and some the reverse. Instead of restlessness and watchfulness, dullness and dejection continue from first to last. Even respiration does not cause embarrassment until shortly before death, when the chest is nearly or quite full of water. The inflammation of the pleura is about the same, as are also the tenderness of the sides, the grunt, and the respiratory murmur. The cough, if it still exists, becomes faint and sore, and now and then causes the before mentioned grunt.

These symptoms usually follow epizootic catarrh, sore throat, or bronchitis.

Remedy.—Hygienic treatment, as in pneumonia; bleeding in acute attacks in vigorous horses and cattle. Emetic and antimonials in animals that vomit. A few doses of aconite tincture or calomel and opium for fever. Salines and antipyretics, as in bronchitis and pneumonia. Potassium iodide and colchicum to promote absorption of inflammatory exudate. Ferric chloride tincture for debility and lack of blood. Digitalis and nux vomica aid removal of fluid. Rugs wrung out of hot water to sides, followed by in-rubbing of mustard, washed off in twenty minutes. Moderate counter-irritation with ammonia and soap liniments. Pain reduced by opium or by morphine hypodermically. Tapping if necessary. (See 'hydrothorax.')

For doses, see pages 13 to 29. For a list of 'antipyretics,' see page 31.

PLEURO-PNEUMONIA.

For description, symptoms, and treatment of this disease, see articles 'Pneumonia' and 'Pleurisy.'

HYDROTHORAX (Water in the Chest),

Is a very common termination of pneumonia with pleurisy. It may also follow compound bronchitis, or it may occur independently, the pleura furnishing the water. In some cases water in the belly and head coexist, accompanied by swelled legs, sheath, belly, &c.

The disease is dangerous, but it is sometimes curable. Tapping the chest with a trocar is sometimes successful. When water does not flow from one side, try the other. Some puncture between the fifth and sixth ribs, some the eighth and ninth, choosing the most dependent parts and the least likely to cause injury. Make an incision through the skin, and then introduce the trocar, with a rotating motion, obliquely and upward as far as it will go, or till water escapes. The stylet must be withdrawn as soon as resistance to the introduction of the trocar is felt. If the hole in the trocar should be stopped up with lymph or other substance, clear it with a probe. When clear and within the cavity, water will flow if there is any in that particular part. The trocar must not be kept in unnecessarily long, as air will penetrate the chest through its orifice. The operation is sometimes repeated several times in the course of treatment. In an unsuccessful case Percivall withdrew ten gallons of water. After death, four days after the operation, there were six gallons more in the chest and a quart in the pericardium.

Symptoms.—Eats daintily; looks disspirited; on the approach of some one, rouses up for a moment only; short, quick, labored respiration, becoming more and more manifest as the chest fills with water. When the chest is nearly full, the horse exerts its utmost power; seldom lies down, but when it does, lies on the side containing the most water, and is soon up again. D'Arboval says the spaces between the ribs are enlarged. The pulse, at first small and quick, becomes accelerated and fainter as the disease advances, till it cannot be felt at all. Horse steps with fore legs wide apart and stiffened; gait often unsteady and reeling; breast, belly and sheath show dropsical swellings, which by degrees fall into the legs.

Auscultation and percussion reveal no sound, unless there is gas or air in the chest, which is rarely the case. Percivall says that if an assistant taps one side of the chest while the surgeon holds his ear to the other, the presence of water may be ascertained. In a recorded and successfully treated case, the sound of the water was comparable to that of water in a rolling cask.

Remedy.—Digitalis; powdered cantharides; potassium nitrate twice daily for a week. Then potassium iodide and iron salts. Pilocarpine useful in human patients. Iodine ointment and rubefacients externally, or insert under the skin of the chest a plug of tow moistened with an irritant. When necessary, tap with trocar or pneumatic aspirator.

BLEEDING FROM THE LUNGS

Is rare. It is dangerous, but the danger depends on the origin, nature, and extent of the case. Plethora, high or very fat condition, and violent work or feats are conducive of bleeding. The membranous tissues, being overcharged with blood, are liable, on extraordinary exertion, to give way; but the bleeding may be owing to over-force of circulation. Wound of the substance of the lung is often the cause of sudden death. It may be caused by violence in hunting, racing, &c., or result from ulceration of the lung in consumption. 'Pulmonic apoplexy' (blood in the air cells) is said to be a dangerous form of lung bleeding.

Symptoms.—When from the bronchial membrane: Blood from *both* nostrils, usually scarlet colored and frothy, attended with more or less irritation, coughing, or snorting and sometimes interrupted breathing; every time the horse coughs or snorts fresh blood is ejected, often through the mouth as well as the nose. The blood does not flow in a uniform stream, as in bleeding from the nose, which is usually from *one* nostril only, and is thus distinguished from bleeding from the lungs, but is influenced by the respiration and also the position of the head and neck; the more the head hangs the readier the blood flows. Sometimes there is febrile disturbance, quick pulse, hot mouth, legs deathly cold, or one cold while another is warm.

Remedy.—Bleeding that cannot be got at, is arrested (1) by cold or heat applied so as to act reflexly; (2) by lead acetate, opium, sulphuric or gallic acid or ferric chloride; (3) hypodermic injection of orgotin.

CONSUMPTION (Tuberculosis, Scrofula, Phthisis),

Is a specific disease, resulting from the introduction into the body of the 'tubercle bacillus.' This mite develops irritation and inflammation, either directly or by the formation of poisonous alkaloids, produced by its action on the tissues. Hard growths appear, consisting of one or more of three descriptions of cell—lymphoid, epitheliod, and giant. They exhibit a tendency to necrosis, followed by caseation (curd or cheese), and occasionally by fibroid degeneration. The disease may be localized in various organs and tissues. It occurs in all animals, and is communicable from one species of animal to another. Cattle, poultry, and hogs are more subject to its several forms than horses, dogs, or sheep. (Dun.) Rare.

Symptoms.—First stage : Out of condition; rough coat; hide bound perhaps; faulty or weak at work; sweats on slight exertion; coughs occasionally after drinking or when first brought out of stable; short-winded. Duration uncertain; weeks, months, and in rare cases years.

Second stage : Case develops itself more or less; respiration probably slightly disturbed; if not perceptible at the flanks or nostrils, apply the ear to the breast or side; by the latter means or by the hand tenderness about the sides may also be discovered; pulse quicker than natural; short, dry cough now and then; appetite fastidious and changeable, now good, now indifferent; never quite lost; spirits same as appetite; sparing issue of yellow matter from nose; flesh lost daily; hip bones begin to project; quarters lose plumpness; skin becoming tense and adherent to sides.

Third stage : Increased disturbance of respiration; the breath, mouth, and discharge from nose fetid; highly quickened pulse; troublesome cough, with occasional coughing up of expectorated matters through the nose and mouth; emaciation and debility; partial separation of coat, so that when but slightly twitched the hair comes off; dropsical swellings perhaps of the legs, sheath, and belly; complete loss of appetite; general irritability; distressing, haggard expression of countenance; irritable state of the bowels and great proneness to diarrhea; the latter is likely to result in death. Breath cold in all stages.

Remedy.—Generous, rather oleaginous diet. Maintain healthy functions of bowels and other excreting organs. No bleeding—not even where there is a tuberculous taint. Milk and flesh liable to transmit the disease to men and animals.

For pulmonary consumption (tuberculosis of lungs)—common in cattle, sheep, and swine: Careful, generous dietary. Good sanitary surroundings. Tonics, acids, alcoholic stimulants, antiseptic inhalations. Arsenic sometimes arrests early stage of consolidation. Iodine liniments and rubefacients externally, also check consolidation and cough. Chloral and morphine relieve cough. (See cough.)

For tuberculous disease of the mesenteric glands: Digestible, nourishing diet. Treat on the same principle as above. Feed off without delay cattle or sheep of tuberculous taint.

For tuberculous abscess of throat or other glands (king's evil): Foment if hot and painful. Dress with iodine liniment. If pus forms, evacuate and treat antiseptically. Liberal dietary, tonics, calcium chloride.

For tubercular arthritis (gouty inflammation), chiefly affecting young animals: Good feeding and sanitation; comfortable quarters. Apply flannels wrung out of hot water or hot oil, followed by mercury oleate and laudanum. Active counter-irritation is injurious.

For doses, see pages 13 to 29.

BROKEN-WIND,

If not asthma, is a sequel of asthma. Its chief cause, according to Williams and Robertson, is eating an undue proportion of hay, especially hay that is overripe, heated, old, dusty, or cut up too short. Robertson says that where " horses are fed on part oat-straw and part hay, both cut rather long, matters are not so bad." Round, shallow-chested horses seem to be predisposed to the disorder.

Williams says broken-wind " is fast becoming a thing of the past."

Symptoms.—Inspiration is easy and rather quick, but expiration is a *double* action, two distinct efforts apparently, after which the muscles relax and the flanks fall peculiarly. Respiratory murmur weakened or absent; loud, sonorous, sibilant wheeze, especially toward back part of chest. Rattling and hissing all over chest; resonance increased, showing that the lungs are distended with air; chest seems rounder, &c.

Cough: It is so peculiar as to be sometimes called " broken-winded cough." It is more than short—it is half-suppressed or chopped off as it were, and so feeble as to be almost inaudible. It is often followed by wheezing, like asthma in man. At first, and also when it afterward comes on in fits, it is troublesome. When the disease is established, and there is no special excitement, it is solitary (but once) as well as short and feeble.

Indigestion: Appetite voracious, yet condition lean and hide-bound looking. Well it may be, for the dung looks like so much chopped hay mixed with oats and husks, causing flatulence and tumid, tense, drum-like belly, often pendent from weakness. Flatulence (expulsion of wind) follows exercise, coughing, dunging, &c., but subsides as the animal relieves itself. In inveterate cases the anus becomes weakened and is as often opened as shut. The interior of the bowel is sometimes exposed, while the anus itself protrudes and recedes with every breath.

Skin: Harsh, dry, and perhaps hide-bound; coat long, rough, and open.

Remedy.—Incurable, but relieved by careful dietary;

good, concentrated food, given damp; water frequently, in limited quantity, but withheld before hard, fast work. Laxatives and salines occasionally. Rock salt, chalk, or whiting in manger. Linseed oil, with lime water, daily, in drench or with food; $\frac{1}{2}$ to 1 grain of arsenic, in the form of Fowler's solution, may be given daily, or every other day, for months. Prof. Dick's cough balls occasionally, consisting of 30 grains each of calomel, opium, digitalis, and camphor. If used daily for a week or more, omit calomel.

For doses, see pages 13 to 29.

SPASM OF THE DIAPHRAGM.

The diaphragm is a large muscle separating the chest from the abdomen. Its spasms are caused by overexertion. It is also sometimes seen in lock-jaw. Its thumpings, sometimes audible at ten paces off, are often confounded with palpitation of the heart. It may be distinguished from the latter (1) by a convulsive movement of the whole body; (2) by difficult breathing; (3) the pulse is small and weak and not synchronous with the beat of the diaphragm; (4) the heart beat is barely perceptible; (5) sometimes profuse sweats and harassing cough.

Remedy.—Quiet; warm clothing. Good, diffusible stimulant. If symptoms continue, give opium. If the difficult breathing is dangerous, moderate bleeding.

For doses, see pages 13 to 29.

Rupture of the diaphragm is common, but is usually perhaps the result of after death swelling. Great internal violence may cause it during life.

Hernia of the diaphragm is like ruptured diaphragm.

DISEASES OF THE STOMACH.

DISEASES of the stomach depend as much perhaps on a lack of mastication and salivary mixture as on the quality or quantity of food. "The food of the horse contains an abundant quantity of starchy materials, and the process by which these are rendered soluble begins in the mouth, not only by their admixture with the salivary secretions, but by a chemical change, through which the non-soluble starch is converted into dextrine and grape sugar, and made fit for the action of the intestinal, biliary, and gastric secretions, and for absorption by the vessels of the intestinal walls. For the purpose of performing this process the horse is provided with 24 millstones in the form of molar teeth. Horses are best kept in health when fed on an admixture of food requiring thorough mastication, and cattle when, in addition to the more nutritious aliments, they are freely supplied with food requiring remastication, such as hay, grass, or straw. An error in the diet or a sudden change from one kind of food to another, not only deranges the stomach, but the intestinal canal as well." (Williams.)

In the horse the process of digestion is only begun in the stomach; it is completed in the intestines. The stomach is small in proportion to the size of the horse; the intestines, in the aggregate, are not. The stomach being small, requires to be often filled. A horse ought not to be worked over five or six hours without food. If it works ten hours, and is given enough food, it is liable to gorge itself. It is also liable, in its haste, to bolt its food.

INFLAMMATION OF THE STOMACH (GASTRITIS),

Is rare as an independent disease. It is probably always the result of irritation of the mucous membrane. This may be caused by improper food, especially in foals and calves; foreign bodies, specific fevers, mineral and vegetable poisons, &c.

Symptoms.—There are no *sure* signs to detect the independent form of the disease. In the poisonous form the symptoms vary with the dose and effect rather than with the kind of poison. Blue vitriol, corrosive sublimate, or arsenic causes nausea, loathing of food, often accompanied by a discharge of saliva; horse paws, looks distressfully at flanks, lies down, rolls about, rises in great agony; quick and painful heaving at the flanks; finally breaks into profuse perspiration. Other poisons cause vomiting, belching, enormous gaseous distension; pulse at first quick, then contracted to a thread, afterward imperceptible; prostration; reels in walking; bowels either violently purged or else so constricted that, notwithstanding painful efforts, nothing but mucus is passed; grows delirious and dangerous; falls, stretches limbs, groans, gapes, dies.

Remedy—An oily laxative removes any irritant and irritant discharges. Ice, with hydrocyanic acid or morphine, or morphine hypodermically, for irritation and pain. Antacids and bismuth, with or without small doses of opium, most useful in young animals. Hot fomentations to abdomen. The brain symptoms and paralysis often occurring in adult cattle, is usually relieved by full doses of oil, followed by demulcents, molasses, salines, and laxative injections. Patients nourished with milk, well boiled gruel, and nutritive clysters. For doses, see pages 13 to 29.

Robertson describes a chronic or mild form of gastritis.

STAGGERS, STOMACH AND GRASS (ACUTE INDIGESTION).

Stomach staggers, according to Robertson, "is chiefly, if not entirely, the result of filling the stomach to repletion." Some foods are worse than others, such as brewers' grain, damaged wheat, ripe vetches, and cooked food. The disorder is not uncommon, and is sometimes very dangerous. In frequency, however, it has fallen off about fifty per cent. in the past sixty years. Cause—regular and judicious feeding. The infrequency of the disorder in France is attributed to the use of laxative and digestible foods. Sleepy, mad, and apoplectic staggers are apparently only conditions or effects of stomach staggers, for severe cases of the latter perhaps always affect the brain more or less.

Grass staggers is caused by rye grass. It paralyzes the limbs, especially the hind limbs, having little if any affect on the brain. Robertson says it is caused by the seed stems of the grass, which horses eat in preference to any other part, and that the time of danger is the ripening time. Cattle and sheep are little affected, for they eat the body of the grass, losing, if they lose any part, the stem. Lambs, however, he says, sometimes suffer, for they nip the stems, but more in play than to obtain food. Williams says the grass is also dangerous when it has been cut and allowed to heat and ferment before being used. Little is positively known about the specific poison in question.

Symptoms.—Stomach staggers: Usually sudden "fugitive abdominal pain;" lies down, but soon up; down again; soon greater restlessness; continued or interrupted pawing; head protruded; in some cases belching; in rare cases attempts at vomiting, with a liquid discharge from the nose. In severe cases acute pain, belching, straining to vomit; lies down carefully.

The sleepy stage (condition) is characterized by dullness;

head hangs; disposed to press it against something; refuses to eat; when forced to change position, shows want of control over movements; disposed to press head against wall again; breathing more or less stertorous.

The mad stage is dangerous; horse liable to do anything. This stage appears to be very rare.

The symptoms of grass staggers develop gradually. Paralysis of hind limbs; in a day or two the weakness increases; reels in walking; danger of falling; disinclined to lie down; anxious countenance; partial paralysis of fore legs; perfect consciousness; calm; bowels rather confined; urine, appetite, breathing, and pulse natural. In severe cases there is the same disposition to stand, even steadying body against wall or stall. Muscular twitchings sometimes occur, and in rare cases brain disturbance; when unable to stand and down, muscular twitchings usually excessive; limbs move automatically; consciousness impaired; breathing stertorous; death near. These symptoms may vary, but chiefly as to rapidity of development or intensity in individual cases.

Remedy.—Aloes or calomel and oil to unload the stomach and bowels. Ether or spirit of ammonia every two hours overcomes flatulence and spasm. Clysters, hand rubbing, exercise. Hot fomentations or cloths wrung out of hot water, or in-rubbing of merely warming dose of mustard, abate spasm and pain. If pain persists, morphine and atrophine hypodermically. One or two doses of aconite tincture sometimes useful. Bleeding sometimes advisable if brain disturbance or breathing occurs. A long, fine trocar and canula in extreme swelling. Strychnine and counter-irritants to spine for paralysis. In young animals, where stomach is overloaded with clots of curd, oil, followed by ether or spirit of ammonia.

For doses, see pages 13 to 29.

DYSPEPSIA (CHRONIC INDIGESTION),

Is a faulty conversion of food into its natural elements. In the horse, owing to the food continuing in the stomach but a comparatively short time, much of the digestive process is performed in the intestines. Indigestion therefore is not altogether the fault of the stomach.

The seat of indigestion seems to be the hair-like or velvet-like lining of the stomach or intestinal canal. These membranes furnish secretions indispensably necessary to the due conversion of food into nourishing and feculent matter, and one or both of them may be functionally faulty, causing irritation, inflammation, &c. But there may be other causes, namely—imperfect mastication and salivary secretion; torpid liver; the bile may be defective in quality or quantity; also the pancreatic juice; or there may be derangement in the worm-like movements of the intestines, by means of which their contents are propelled.

The disorder is peculiar to young horses, especially such as are reared in low, marshy, cold, poor pastures. The coarse, rank, sour grass seems to lay the foundation of disease of the bowels.

Symptoms.—The symptoms are plain, but it is usually difficult to name the part or organ that is affected. The horse is dull and spiritless, though the appetite may be even voracious; but it may be intermittent—good at one time, bad at another; sometimes it is depraved, horse eating dirt, plaster, brick, wood, stones, &c.; coat penfeathered, dry, and perhaps scurfy, nor is it shed at the usual season; hide-bound; dung either darker or lighter than natural, with offensive odor, and coated with mucus; when broken, crumbles to pieces, appearing to consist of loosely compacted chopped hay, mingled with many entire or imperfectly dissolved oats; colicky pains in severe or advanced cases; inclined to be costive when in stable, but exercise causes purging; skin sympathizes, as shown by the coat; it may be in a morbid or perhaps eruptive condition.

Remedy.—Careful dietary; avoid long fasts; vary food; water at reasonable intervals, or keep it in stable constantly. A laxative is almost invariably the first requisite, conjoined with a cholagogue in bilious cases. (Cholagogues promote the flow of bile. See 'Purgatives,' page 35.) Alkalies, chalk, magnesia before feeding, or with food in debilitated cases. Ball of whiting and piece of rock salt in rack. Alkalies may be conjoined with nux vomica and other bitters. Hydrochloric or other mineral acids, with bitters and iron salts, preferable to alkalies in persistent cases. Hard worked horses often benefited by mixing an ounce of linseed oil with food daily. Glycerine, especially for young. Ox-bile with gentian or nux vomica in intractable cases. Bismuth and hydrocyanic acid in chronic gastric irritability. Creosote, eucalyptus, peppermint oils for undue fermentation. Arsenic with morphine in chronic irritable cases, and where food causes diarrhea.

For doses, see pages 13 to 29.

BOTS (Afterward Gad-Flies),

Are little grub-like creatures, voided with the dung. As a rule they are not injurious. In some cases, however, when present in large numbers, they are injurious, and may cause, or at least aid in causing, death. It is said that no known medicine will destroy the bot while in the stomach.

The gad-fly or bot undergoes about as many transformations as the butter-fly. The egg is deposited on the hair in autumn, is conveyed to the tongue by licking, hatched by the heat and moisture almost instantly, and is then conveyed, with the food, to the stomach, where it remains during the winter, its dark-brown hooks being securely fixed in the cuticular coat, a part that is said to be as insensible to pain as are the hoofs. In the spring it releases its hold, is conveyed to the intestines, and sooner or later expelled. It dries, assumes a crysalis state for about two months, and then is born as a gad-fly.

Remedy.—Turpentine and oils, bitters, hydrochloric acid, copper and iron sulphates, arsenic; then purgatives. Green fodder. Destroy larvæ and fly.

For doses, see pages 13 to 29.

RUPTURE OF STOMACH

Is a natural though not necessary termination of unrelieved gorged stomach, and perhaps also chronic indigestion or other disease. It may also be caused by the strain of vomiting, or attempted vomiting, the struggles of the horse while suffering, stones in the stomach, external violence, &c. It is peculiar to old and exhausted horses. Fatal. Morphine injected under the skin will afford some relief.

FLATULENT STOMACH (COLIC),

Is caused by the stomach or intestines, or both, becoming distended with air or gas (gas from food). The disorder is usually caused by green food—grass, wheat, rye, &c. The condition of the stomach is sometimes an important factor. Crib-biters are predisposed to colic. A sharp trot will often give a crib-biter relief.

Remedy.—See 'Colic, Spasmodic and Flatulent,' pages 102, 103, 104.

POLYPUS (TUMOR) OF STOMACH.

Dr. Brown describes one, weighing $7\frac{1}{4}$ ounces, that apparently caused no inconvenience till it obstructed the pylorus. It had a rather tortuous pedicle, 3 inches long by 1 in diameter, with an artery and 2 veins in its center. About 15 inches of "the first small gut were mortified."

DISEASES OF THE INTESTINES

The intestines are more subject to disease than the stomach. They are of far greater bulk, the part they perform in the process of digestion is more complex, and the aliment remains in them much longer, so that anything hurtful it may contain has a better chance to develop itself. Further, owing to their great length, tortuosities, and difference in shape and size, concretions are more likely to form within and obstruct them. Again, owing to their worm-like movements, one is liable to get twisted or knotted, which may cause death. Some intestinal diseases are acute and rapid in their course; others are so mild and insidious that they are not noticed—or, if noticed, not till it is too late. Remedies must be given promptly.

SPASMODIC COLIC

Is caused by spasm or cramp of some part or parts of the intestinal tube. The tube, by means of its muscular coat, possesses self-contracting power, which enables it to propel its contents onward from the stomach. When the contraction is such as to cause spasm or cramp, spasmodic colic follows. The tube is usually contracted to a third or a fourth or more of its natural diameter, and at intervals of two, three, or four inches. Sometimes they are one, two, or three feet apart. The usual seat of cramp is the small intestines, but the large ones are not exempt.

According to Gamgee, who is corroborated by Williams, colic is caused by an irritant in the intestinal canal, and is best treated by purgatives and injections. Pain and spasm are only symptoms.

The causes are over and irregular feeding—even with healthy food; cooked foods and foods of bad quality; too much rye, wheat, vetches, peas, and other green foods; sudden changes of food; overdrinking when heated; disease of, and parasites, poisons, and stones in, the intestines; diseases of contiguous parts; the influence of cold and damp on the surface of the body, &c.

Ordinary cases are relieved by a single dose of medicine—sometimes without medicine. In severe cases if relief does not come in about six hours, recovery is doubtful. Fatal cases usually terminate in about 24 hours. Whatever is given must be given at once. Watch for relapses.

Stallions should be examined for symptoms of rupture. Examine the scrotum; also the inguinal (groin) canals and abdominal rings. (See 'Inguinal Hernia,' page 58.)

Spasmodic colic is distinguished from inflammation of the bowels (enteritis) in many ways, namely: there is no preceding indisposition; no cold, hot, or shivering fits; expressions of pain are stronger, and come on by fits and starts; remissions of pain, but constant watchfulness, as if in expectation of pain; pulse contracted to a thread, yet not exceeding 50; drops down suddenly and rolls about, instead of lying down quietly; absence of heat about the abdomen.

Symptoms.—Attack sudden; paws, stamps, and strikes belly with hind feet; after bending knees and crouching body several times, advances hind feet in attempts to lie down; at last drops rather than lies down, the fall causing a grunt; rolls, each time trying to balance on its back; if, by getting against the stall, it succeeds, remains quiet for a minute or two, the feet drawn down to the belly, the head and neck curved to one side perhaps. Sometimes, if it fails to balance on its back, it will rise suddenly, shake itself, and stand quietly for a time. But it soon averts its head and looks at its flanks anxiously.

Fit follows fit, each one usually increasing in length and severity, the intervals of ease being imperceptible; physical exertion and convulsions cause profuse perspiration; drops of sweat stand on the brows and eyelashes.

The next state is one of delirium, violence, danger; eyes wild; cold sweats; tremors; falls, or perhaps from the maddening pain, throws itself down and dies.

The pulse at first and during remissions of pain is little altered; during pain, as before said, it quickens and is contracted to a thread, being at times almost imperceptible; during extreme pain, its quickness and perceptibility are increased; belly tense, sometimes swollen, and usually very tender; bowels constipated, though dung will often pass on the eve of an attack, and sometimes afterward; also urine.

Remedy.—See 'Flatulent Colic.'

FLATULENT COLIC

Is not as common as 'spasmodic colic,' but it is more dangerous. It is caused by indigestion, foods which easily undergo fermentation, such as raw potatoes, green clover, brewers' grain, wheat, and boiled food, crib-biting, &c. It may follow spasmodic colic. Its seat is the large intestines—cæcum and colon.

Symptoms.—Unlike spasmodic colic, there are no remissions of pain, and the belly is more or less tensely swollen and resonant on percussion; pulse soon becomes rapid and feeble; breathing rapid and mostly thoracic (belonging to the chest); extremities cold; more or less delirium; reels to and fro; muscles twitch; lips retracted, &c.

Remedy.—Purgative to remove irritant; aloes for the horse, oils and salines for cattle and sheep. Purgation hastened and pain relieved by copious laxative clyster injections, hot fomentations, friction to abdomen, and gentle exercise. Ether, oil of turpentine, other volatile oils, ammonia and ammonium carbonate combat flatulence. Ether, alcohol, and chloral hydrate, with opium, belladonna, or cannabis indica, control spasm and pain. Morphine and atrophine hypodermically promptly relieve spasm. Inhalation of chloroform quiets violent spasmodic cases.

Repeated recurring attacks in influenza, often connected

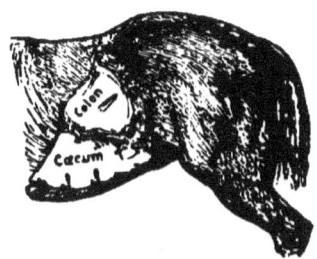

Fig. 19. Where to puncture for Flatulent Colic.

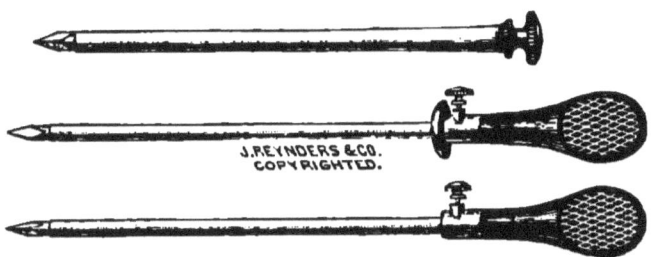

Fig. 20. Cæcum and Colon Trocars.

with liver disease, treated with half dose of aloes and a little calomel, spirit of chloroform and mustard in-rubbing to abdomen

In intractable 'Flatulent Colic,' trocar colon.

For doses, see pages 13 to 29.

INFLAMMATION OF THE BOWELS (ENTERITIS),

Is the most rapidly fatal disease perhaps to which the horse is subject, causing death sometimes in a few hours. According to Williams, it is more like an apoplexy than an inflammation. Robertson says it is different from ordinary inflammations both in its clinical and after-death features. The large as well as the small bowels are liable to attack, the weakest or most irritated parts suffering first probably.

Its most frequent causes perhaps are overfatigue, cold from exposure, washing with very cold water while heated and afterward inadequately clothed, overfeeding previous to hard work, injuries to the intestines, and certain diseases. It is liable, in some cases, to settle in the feet, especially the fore feet. Examine stallions for rupture. Pressure of the abdomen is a good test for enteritis; but the surest test is examination per rectum with the oiled hand.

Recoveries are rare, death resulting either from mortification or hemorrhage—blood in the colon or other intestine.

The disease is distinguished from spasmodic colic (1) by the pulse, which is full, firm, and accelerated to double or treble its natural frequency; (2) history of case; (3) manner of attack—not so sudden; (4) intermissions—practically none; (5) progress of case.

Symptoms.—No appetite; dull and feverish; paws, stamps, strikes belly, cringes, &c., very much as in spasmodic colic; paws with one foot for hours; anxious and painful expression of eye; belly tense, painful, and drawn up toward flanks; dung hard, angular, and dark colored. As the disease progresses, animal becomes restless, breathes hard, sighs, perhaps snorts; breathing sooner or later becomes hurried as well as hard; nostrils dilated; countenance painfully vigilant; bathed in sweat—one time hot, another cold; occasional tremor; tail erect and quivering; mouth hot and dry; pulse 80 to 120—hard, wiry.

The last stage borders on delirium; wild, haggard stare, pupils dilating; danger. Suddenly a change comes—the change of mortification; pain ceases; quiet; drinks and attempts to eat; breathing tranquil, but breath more or less fetid; pulse imperceptible; cold, clammy sweat; tremor from head to foot; ears, legs, mouth deadly cold; little dung has passed. Convulsions return. Death.

Sometimes the symptoms at first are comparatively mild. They indicate mechanical obstruction perhaps.

Remedy.—Morphine and atrophine hypodermically at intervals of 2 hours for bloody effusion. Ergotin has been conjoined with these with view of contracting blood vessels. Half dram each of opium, belladonna extract, and camphor in pint of gruel every 2 hours. Where heart action is violent, 10 to 15 minims B. P. tincture aconite may be added. Bleeding sometimes useful in early stages in vigorous subjects. No purging. Laxative injections. From the first apply rugs wrung out of hot water around trunk for 2 hours. Then rub belly with soap liniment and opium (opium in liniment).

Enteritis is not as sudden in other animals as in the horse, nor so rapidly fatal. Bleed robust subjects. Few doses of aconite, or oil and calomel. Hot fomentations, mustard, and soap liniment. For doses, see pages 13 to 29.

DIARRHEA

May be independent, or it may be the result of some other disorder. When independent, it is simply an effort of nature to rid itself of unhealthy matter. This is well, even if it is caused by green food. But it must not go too far, for diarrhea may be followed by dysentery. Long continuance in cold, wet, rank pastures sometimes has this result.

Diarrhea may result from increased peristaltic (wormlike) action of the bowels, congestion or inflammation of their mucous membrane, disorder of the liver, mesenteric glands, intestinal worms, &c. Too much cold water just before work, or during work, is bad. Some waters seem to possess diarrheal properties.

Diarrhea in foals and calves is often attended with serious or fatal results, and it is sometimes epizootic. Its cause is functional disturbance, which is intimately associated with the process of digestion.

Remedy.—Laxatives in first stage to remove irritant. Rest; comfortably warm. Restrict water; diet carefully; wheaten flour gruel. Alkalies; chalk where dejections (excrements or feces) are acid. Mineral acids or gallic acid, with opium, in profuse watery discharges. Injections of starch gruels at 100° F., with lead acetate and opium. Aromatics and camphor abate nervous irritability. Oil of cinnamon in cases resulting from cold. Volatile oils, ether, chloroform, chlorodyne in moderate but frequently repeated doses relieve flatulence and spasm. Ammonia carbonate where watery secretions are continued and the heart action weak. Arsenic and opium in chronic cases. Copper sulphate; corrosive sublimate, with creosote and opium, when chronic discharges contain mucus and blood. Ergotin and opium, with keratin, where the discharges are profuse and continued. Antiseptics, sulphites, sulpho-carbolates where discharges are foul. Nitric acid and nux vomica when complicated with liver disorder.

For young animals: Castor oil with a few drops laudnum. While patient is fed on milk, if it disagrees when given with lime water in cautiously regulated, restricted quantity, substitute cooked starch food, or beef tea and white of egg, with a little wine or spirit, if the animal is reduced. Gray powder where the discharge is pale and fetid. (For doses, see pages 13 to 29.) 'Spirit' usually means alcohol; but it also means whisky, gin, wine, &c.

DYSENTERY OR BLOODY FLUX

Is comparatively rare, but dangerous. It consists in inflammation and ulceration of the mucous membrane and glandular structures of the large and sometimes the small intestines, and is attended with fever, occasional abdominal pain, fluid discharges, mingled with blood or albuminous materials (floating, coffee-ground-like lumps). It resembles diarrhea in several of its features, and sometimes follows it. It is caused by bad food and water and exposure in low, wet, marshy pastures, the filth and malaria of overcrowded stables, blood contamination, intestinal parasites, &c.

The disease is best differentiated from diarrhea by the character of the bowel discharges. These contain a moderate quantity of true fecal matter, either soft or hard. The liquid part is composed largely of mucus and a jelly-like material, mingled with shreds of membrane or blood, the whole being of a tenacious, gluey character, and emitting a peculiarly offensive smell.

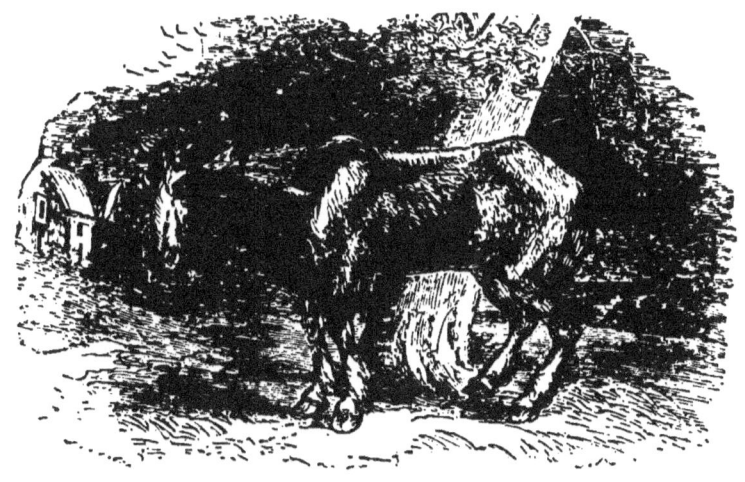

Fig. 21. Chronic Dysentery.

Remedy.—Digestible, soft food; restricted water supply; quiet. Small occasional doses gray powder or calomel, with other antiseptics. Occasional dose of castor oil and laudanum for fever. Lead acetate and opium, gallic, tannic, or mineral acids, with opium, or carbolized glycerine and opium, in solution, or bolus incased in keratin.

Chloroform, chlorodyne, with opium, relieve tenesmus (inability to dung). Opium as anodyne—by mouth, injection, and suppository. (For doses, see pages 13 to 29.)

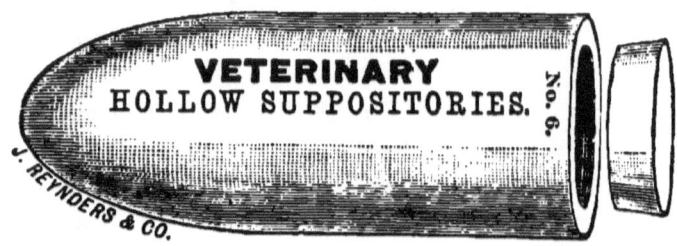

Fig. 22. Suppository. One of these Suppositories, filled with wet tobacco, and inserted in the rectum, will usually cure colic in a few minutes. The same treatment will destroy 'pin worms' in horses, say Reynders & Co.

CONSTIPATION

May exist independently or be the result of a disease or a combination of diseases. The independent form, which is rarely dangerous, is usually the result of lack of bowel motion, fluid material, green or soft food, &c.

Symptoms.—Weakness; disturbed appetite; hair long; skin dry; legs disposed to swell; often pot-bellied; pulse sometimes small, weak, and perhaps accelerated; mouth fetid; mucous membranes and tongue soapy; in bad cases lips and gums may be covered with dark, pus-and-blood-like matter, &c.

Remedy.—Laxative diet, diluents, salines, regular exercise. Moderate purgatives, especially in liver disorder; laxative clysters. Aloes, oils, calomel, small doses Epsom salt for horses. Epsom salt, croton, gamboge, calomel for cattle. Gentian, quinine and other tonics for debilitated. Oil of turpentine by mouth and rectum for flatulence. Soap suppository in young animals. Nux vomica, belladonna, physostygmine in chronic cases. Electricity and ergot give tone.

Where stones or twisted intestines cause the obstruction,

avoid purgatives. Use diluents, laxative injections, and anodynes. (For doses, see pages 13 to 29.)

INTESTINAL AND STOMACH CONCRETIONS (CALCULI),

Are divided by Prof. Morton into phosphatic, oat-hair, and mixed. The phosphatic are hard, smooth, and polished, having hard substances (stones, &c.) for nuclei (centers); the oat-hair are larger but less dense, having beards of oats, barley, &c., for nuclei; the mixed are composed of phosphatic salts, oat-hair, and fecal and indigestible matter. They vary in size from mere pebbles to large stones—even 25 pounds. The impassable stones cause irritation and sometimes death. When within reach they may be removed per rectum. Sift the food. Phosphatic foods and hard water are factors.

Remedy.—Explore rectum; use long injection tube. Avoid active purgatives. Morphine and atrophine hypodermically for spasm and pain.

For doses, see pages 13 to 29.

WORMS (INTESTINAL).

Four kinds are peculiar to the horse. 1. The 'Ascaris lumbricoides,' resembling the common earth worm, inhabits the small intestines. It is round, nearly as large as the little finger, and varies in length from three or four inches to a foot or even two feet. It is white or reddish-white in color. Usually only one is passed at a time, but 150 have been known to pass in a week. Chabert found 14 pounds in one horse.

2. The 'Ascaris vermicularis,' a lively, needle-like worm, inhabits the large intestines. It is perhaps the most pernicious of the four kinds. It is from one-half to three inches long. The head is obtuse, the tail sharp pointed. There is a semi-transparent and a black variety.

3. The 'Strongylus' is similar in size to the red worm

used by fishermen. It is from two to four inches long, and has two distinct parts—body and tail. The tail is thread-like, and constitutes more than half the worm's length. When first voided, they appear black, the tail and sometimes the head being transparent. When taken from the dung, they vomit up their black contents and die.

4. The 'Tænia' (tape-worm) is white, flat, thin, broad, and jointed at regular intervals. It is said to sometimes measure twenty feet in length. The head, which is tuberculous and attached to the smaller end of the body, is said to be directed toward and sometimes within the stomach. They are rare.

The worms are rarely numerous enough to cause death, but when present in large numbers they cause more or less harm. They die shortly after the horse dies. Poverty of body, insufficient nutrition, stagnant water, and miasms are said to be conducive of them. They are peculiar to young horses.

Symptoms.—Colicky pains; attempts to dung, but little passes except glairy mucus; oscillatory motion of the tail; rubbing root of tail, owing to itching about anus; white or yellow powder about anus; depraved and fastidious appetite; fond of salt; rubbing upper lip; coat dry and rough, remaining in patches long after shedding time; hide-bound; lean and unable to thrive; feverish; pulse small and quick; mouth unusually dry and warm. But the best sign is the worm itself.

Remedy.—Aloes, oil turpentine, bitters. Ferric chloride, copper sulphate. Aconite tincture, salt in manger.

Oil turpentine and male shield fern for tape-worm.

For doses, see pages 13 to 29.

TWISTED OR STRANGLED BOWELS (VOLVULUS),

Is usually caused by the worm-like movements of the long, loose, and coiled intestines, but a long-necked tumor, by winding itself around the intestine, may cause the same result—strangling. The symptoms resemble those of inflammation of the bowels. Rupture of the intestine may result, but the disease is usually fatal whether it does or not.

Remedy.—It cannot be rectified by medical treatment, but a surgical operation, if undertaken early, may be successful.

INTUSSUSCEPTION OR INTROSUSCEPTION

Is the slipping of a part of one intestine into another, usually the one behind. Cartwright reports a case of 12 introsusceptions, and another where a foot of intestine was invaginated. Walker reports a case of 2 feet; Turner one of 16 feet 4 inches; Hales found the whole of the cæcum within the colon, and inverted at that.

The symptoms resemble those of inflammation of the bowels, but there are intermissions of pain; also sighing, groaning, lying on the belly, resting on the hind quarters, and a disposition, when down, to stay down. Usually fatal.

Remedy.—No treatment is of much avail. Restrict to a limited quantity of soft food. No purging. Opium and cannabis indica allay spasm and pain. Prof. Smith's long enema tube may be tried.

For doses, see pages 13 to 29.

PILES (HEMORRHOIDS),

Is rare in the horse. It is peculiar to dogs, and is the result of congestion of the mucous membrane around the anus and dilatation of the hemorrhoidal veins.

Remedy.—Oily aperients, laxative injections. Remove hardened dung. Return prolapsed bowel. Cooling, digestible diet. Gall and opium ointment, or zinc benzoate ointment.

For doses, see pages 13 to 29.

PROTRUSION OF THE ANUS OR RECTUM

Is rare.

Remedy.—Return the bowel carefully, first washing with dilute alcohol, laudanum, and a little carbolic acid. Close external opening with truss or stitches. Control straining by opium or chloral. When the rectum is much swollen, scarify carefully.

For doses, see pages 13 to 29.

DISEASES OF THE URINARY ORGANS.

The kidney is a very susceptible organ. It is easily affected by medicine, a fact of great importance to practitioners. Sometimes medicines given as purges, instead of acting on the bowels, apparently expend their whole force on the kidneys, giving the urine, which is copious, a dark color. This fact probably accounts for mercury being so slow in producing salivation.

A case of *single* kidney, but of double size, is recorded.

The urine may contain excess of water, urea, coloring matter, and inorganic constituents; also a deficiency of water and inorganic constituents. There may be alteration of other organic compounds, the acid constituents and extractive matters. It may contain albumen, bile compounds, sugar, blood, pus, mucus, calculi, &c. It is naturally alkaline in herb-eating and acid in flesh-eating animals. It differs in composition in various animals, but some of its constituents are identical.

INFLAMMATION OF THE KIDNEYS (NEPHRITIS),

Is rare. It is usually caused by medicinal irritation—turpentine, the resins, cantharides (internal or blister), croton oil, &c.; stimulating food, cold, water dripping on the back and loins, injuries, &c. Robertson describes two forms. He also describes kidney congestion.

Symptoms.—There are many, but the surest are scanty secretion or total suppression of urine; frequent attempts to stale, passing perhaps but a few drops of highly colored, unhealthy urine. In the stallion retraction (drawing back) of the testicle on the affected side may be present. The symptoms are sometimes indicative of colic rather than kidney disease.

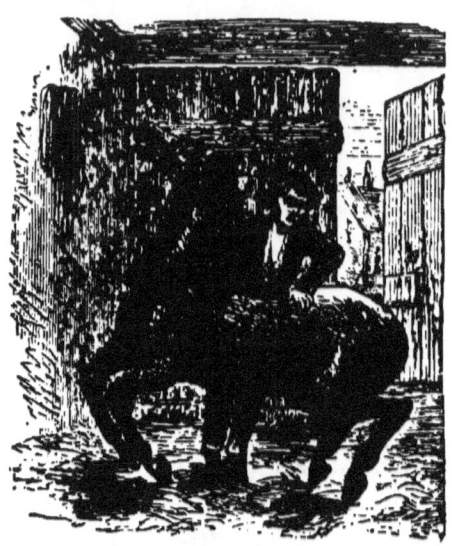

Fig. 23. The test for Inflammation of the Kidneys.

Remedy.—Bleeding if febrile symptoms acute. Aconite in early stages of acute cases. Gentle laxatives remove waste products and lessen work of kidneys. In suppression of urine, digitalis decoction repeatedly applied to loins. Linseed, diluents, barley water. Promote skin functions. Alkaline bicarbonates and sulphites as antiseptics. Anodyne clysters relieve reflexly. Fomentations or fresh sheep skins to loins. Where chronic irritation remains, belladonna, opium, camphor as anodynes.

For doses, see pages 13 to 29.

ALBUMINOUS URINE (ALBUMINURIA),

Is rare. It is best determined perhaps by chemical tests. Tested with bichloride of mercury, it yields a copious milky precipitate. If it does not coagulate on exposure to heat, add acetic acid, and then prussiate of potash.

According to Percivall and Williams, the following are more or less constant

Symptoms.—Standing with distended legs, perhaps all day, not for staling, but for comfort; or standing "all of a heap," back roached, hind legs advanced. When led, back and loins stiff; some fever. In severe cases there are rigors, accelerated respiration, loud puffing at nostrils, anxious countenance, small, quick pulse, disinclination to move, pain in turning, and usually constipation.

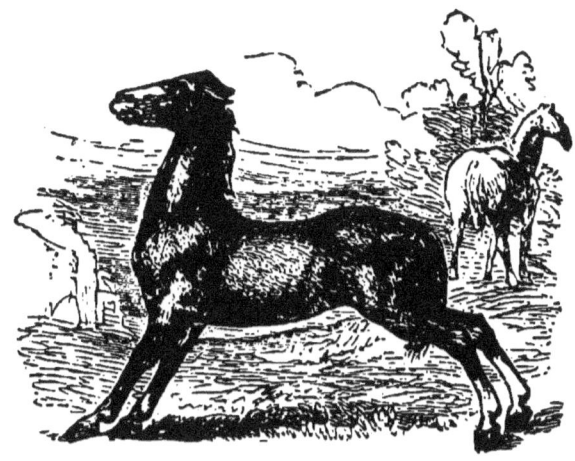

Fig. 24. Positions assumed when suffering from Albuminous Urine.

Remedy.—When it arises from other than kidney disease, it will cease when the cause is removed. When depending on kidney disease, the treatment is only palliative. Aid kidneys by keeping bowels relaxed with good food; keep skin warm; avoid cold; tonics or mineral acids; light work. (Williams.) For list of tonics, see page 37.

BLOOD IN THE URINE (HÆMATURIA),

May appear as bright fluid blood, mixed with the urine, or it may contain a brown or dark colored deposit—blood corpuscles, existing in entirety or undergoing a change. When due to the bladder, it usually follows staling; when from the urethra, it both precedes and succeeds it. It may be caused by external as well as internal injury, disease, strains, overwork, &c.

Remedy.—Oleaginous laxatives; sulphuric acid; iron salts; lead acetate internally. Ergotin and belladonna hypodermically. Fresh sheep skins to loins; spinal hot water bag. For doses, see pages 13 to 29.

URINARY STONES (CALCULI),

Are called 'renal' when in the kidney; 'uretal' when in the tube leading from the kidney to the bladder; 'cystic' or 'vesical' when in the bladder; 'urethral' when in the tube leading from the bladder outward.

Kidney stones usually lodge in the pelvis (cavity) of the kidney, but the funnels or canals are also sometimes filled with them. Like other calculi they differ in size, conformation, and consistence. Some weigh 25 ounces.

Uretal stones are rare. They may be felt per rectum, and may be cut out.

Bladder stones are somewhat common. There are more or less distinct symptoms of their presence, but the best way to decide whether they exist or not is to feel per rectum or vagina, especially when the bladder is empty. The operation is easy and safe. Mares have been known, in their agony, to expel their stones.

Urethral stones are somewhat rare. They are usually as large as a walnut, and hence cannot pass entirely through the canal. They can be felt per rectum, and sometimes, when near the external orifice of the penis, can be touched with the finger.

Remedy.—Dilute mineral acids for horse. Alkalies or alkaline bicarbonates diminish tendency to urinary deposits, common especially among highly fed rams and wethers. Ammonia benzolate helps resolution of phosphatic deposits in sheep. Diluents; cooling, laxative foods. Raise feeding sheep thrice daily and drive them a few hundred yards, to insure urination. Place sheep on buttocks; the sandy deposits in the urethra are gradually moved by manipulation. Where the canal is hopelessly blocked, it must be opened either at the ischial arch or by amputation of the penis. Lithotomy (cutting for stone) in the horse and ox and lithotripsy (triturating or powdering) in mare or cow, the only means of removing large cystic stones.

For doses, see pages 13 to 29.

INFLAMMATION OR CATARRH OF THE BLADDER (CYSTITIS),

Is usually caused (1) by foreign bodies, such as calculi and morbid growths; (2) by irritating medicines—cantharides, &c.; (3) retention of urine.

Symptoms.—Restlessness; paddling or repeated moveing of the hind feet; occasional whisking of tail; frequent discharge of urine in small quantities; pain on examining bladder per rectum; in severe and long-standing cases, where the contractile power of the sphincter is lessened, there may be continuous dribbling of urine; sometimes more or less constitutional disturbance and fever; sometimes subacute or chronic cases, which are often indicated by pus and other cell structures in the urine.

Remedy.—Oleaginous laxatives, aconite, calomel abate fever. Bleeding, followed by above sedatives, in early stages, for acute pain and fever. Belladonna, internally in clyster, and suppository in vagina, for irritation. Softening anodyne injections; hyoscyamus, opium. Rugs wrung out of boiling water, or fresh sheep skins to loins. Mashes, linseed, boiled barley, diluents. Potassium bicarbonate, or other alkalies internally when urine is acid or acrid. Benzoic or boric acid, sulphites, borax, sulphocarbolates, eucalyptus oil when urine alkaline, fermenting, or fetid. Syringe female bladder with alkaline solutions when urine acrid; when fetid, with boro-glycerine or dilute copper sulphate. Buchu, bearberry, eucalyptus in chronic vesical catarrh.

For doses, see pages 13 to 29.

Suppression and Retention of Urine.—Suppression signifies non-secretion of urine; retention inability to pass urine. Suppression of urine may result from inflammation of the kidneys, or anything else that prevents the performance of their functions. Retention of urine may result from spasm or contraction of the neck of the bladder, the lodgment of stones, paralysis, &c. (Percivall.)

See 'Nephritis' and 'Cystitis.'

Cysts in the Kidneys are not rare. A fibrous cyst, as large as a fist, discovered by Percivall, contained eight ounces of black fluid. The fluid was composed of the different elements of the blood, particularly the coloring matter. Usually, however, they contain simply the watery parts of the blood.

Enlargement of the Kidneys (one or both) is not unusual. In a recorded case one kidney weighed 24 lbs., the other 27. In another case the right kidney "was supposed to weigh upward of 112 lbs." The left was healthy, though rather larger than natural.

Inversion and Protrusion of the Bladder sometimes occurs in foaling. If the protruded parts cannot be reduced and returned, perhaps a ligature may be successfully used. Send for a veterinarian.

DISEASES OF THE ORGANS OF GENERATION.

THE diseases of the organs of generation, especially those of the male, are rare in this country and England. Cause—castration. They are also rare in non-breeding females.

A disease—called by the French 'Maladie du Coit' (a disease of copulation)—much resembling syphilis in man, broke out in De Witt county, Illinois, in 1884, the probable cause of which being an imported and infected French stallion. The disease made its way to Kent county, Ontario, Canada, in 1887. Great effort was and is being made to stamp it out. It is as poisonous apparently as glanders-farcy. It is sometimes followed by one or other form of this disease (described on page 67).

EQUINE SYPHILIS (MALADIE DU COIT),

Is a specific equine constitutional disease, characterized by lesions of the urino-genital organs, and communicable from coition by either affected horse or mare. (Dun.)

It is caused by filth, fatty concretions beneath the prepuce, foreign substances within the sheath or urethra, acrid injections into the urethra, accidents, violence in copulation, &c. (D'Arboval.)

The disease usually begins at the head of the penis, extending upward sometimes as far as the lining of the sheath. At first the parts are tense, shining, and painful, but as soon as any morbid tissue appears, the lubrefactive secretion becomes augmented, thickened, and fetid. Sometimes it is mixed with a whitish whey, when the skin of the penis peels off in flakes. Sometimes the disease consists of small, circumscribed, red patches. These are succeeded by or converted into little bladders, which, bursting, leave chancre-like ulcers. When the disease spreads to the urethra, it causes a communicable discharge from it. (D'Arboval.)

The mare, usually in eight or nine days, exhibits uterine excitement resembling exaggerated sexual heat. The vulva becomes swollen; the mucous membrane of the vulva and vagina is reddened; there is a white, yellow, grayish, or reddish vaginal discharge, at first of a watery nature, which soon increases, becoming thicker, sticky, and viscid, collecting about and soiling the tail and perinæum. (W. L. Williams.)

Dr. Williams, whose experience is confined to the Illinois outbreak, calls the disease 'Equine Syphilis.' It is very insidious at first in the stallion, and is besides very deceptive—appearing to be cured when it is not. Of its many bad effects, the worst perhaps is paralysis of the hind quarters.

According to most authorities there is a benign form of the disease. M. Rodloff says that the benign and malignant forms are distinct diseases, and that the former never appears with the latter except by accident.

Remedy.—Mucilaginous and anodyne vaginal injections allay irritation in the mare in the early stages. Follow with astringent injections of zinc or copper sulphates or silver nitrate. Treat male with similar astringents. Cast. The blood being very deficient in fibrin, French veterinarians prescribe bouillon of ox blood and horse flesh. Crushed oats and beans should also be serviceable. (Dun.)

For doses, see pages 13 to 29.

Many months often elapse before cure is effected. In Prussia stallions are not allowed to be used till three years after recovery.

INFLAMMATION OF THE MEMBRANE OF THE PENIS (BALANITIS),

Is contagious, especially when of a specific or impure form.

Remedy.—Zinc sulphate or lead subacetate, diluted solutions. Zinc oxide ointment. Laxative. Anodyne injections. Chronic specific cases, often caused by leucorrhea in female, accompanied by effusion and pain, require scarification and continued fomentation. Horse or bull must be cast and secured. Inflamed ulcerated surfaces dressed with zinc oxide ointment, carbolized, or mercuric nitrate ointment. Quiet and rest; dose of physic. Laxative diet. For doses, see pages 13 to 29.

INFLAMMATION OF THE URETHRA (URETHRITIS),

Is rare, being peculiar to stallions. Its causes are: Too frequent acts of copulation; copulation with a female having inflammation of the vagina, or a vagina small in proportion to the male organ; irritation of the alimentary canal, caused by drenches, balls of cantharides, &c., given to reinvigorate the stallion; irritation of worms in the rectum; shifting of irritation; inflammation in the bladder; retention of urine. (D'Arboval.)

Symptoms.—Horse, in act of staling, looks at flanks, stamps, switches tail, moaning and showing uneasiness when through; urethra red, swollen, and moist from discharge. In a few days stales oftener, with increase of pain and swelling; discharge increases, grows thicker, turns yellow or green; it may be squeezed out, causing streaks of blood perhaps; frequent and painful erections; penis grows curved; engorgement of testicles, spermatic cords, scrotum, sheath; testicles hang lower, sometimes swell, growing hard and painful, especially the oblong attachment called the epididymis; spermatic cord sympathizes and presents a mushroom-like aspect; exterior ulcers and buds on and near lower part of penis; sometimes red, exuberant granulations also. (D'Arboval.)

Remedy.—Copper, zinc, or silver salts injected in dilute solution, 1 part to 60 of water. Oils of copaiba and eucalyptus internally and locally. Prevent occlusion (closing)

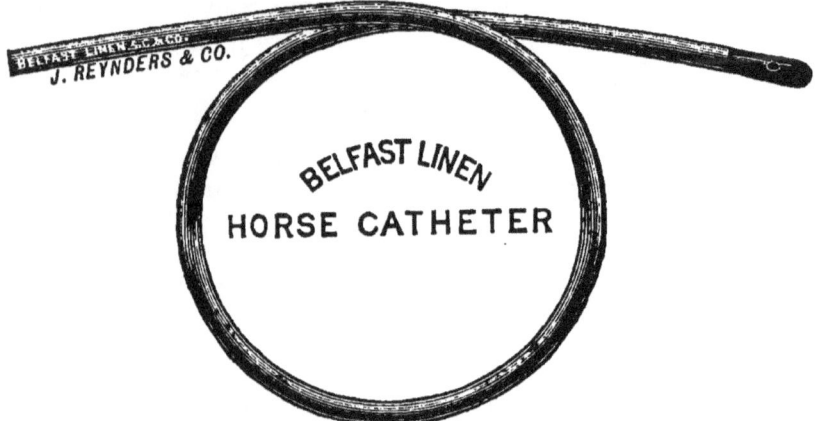

Fig. 25. Catheter.

by cautious introduction of catheter. Persistent obstruction in male, from inflammation or gravel, sometimes requires perineal opening. For doses, see pages 13 to 29.

INFLAMMATION AND CATARRH (LEUCORRHEA) OF THE VAGINA.

Acute inflammation, in the absence of injury, is rare. In catarrh the discharge is sometimes whey-like, sometimes yellow and even purulent; often, in both cases, becoming thin, clear, and water-like. The discharge collects and comes away every time the lips of the vulva open with a sort of gush. In general there is not much, if any, reddening of the inside of the vagina.

Remedy.—Siphon or syringe the uterus and vagina with tepid alkaline solutions, and subsequently with dilute carbolic acid or zinc sulphate. Belladonna or iodoform in suppository, or injection where there is excessive secretion or pain. (See Fig. 22.) Copper or iron salts, turpentine internally, especially in delicate subjects or in obstinate recurring cases associated with tuberculosis.

For doses, see pages 13 to 29.

INFLAMMATION OF THE WOMB (METRITIS),

Is rare in the mare. It is usually caused by foaling, and is accompanied by bloody discharges. Other symptoms resemble colic and inflammation of the bowels, but the suffering is not so great. It is common in cows and ewes, and is liable to spread by contagion. The inflammation sometimes extends to the peritoneum.

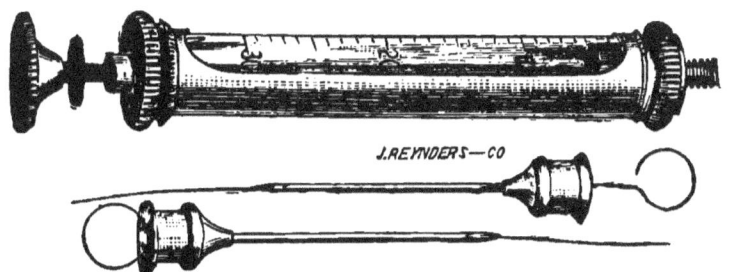

Fig. 26. Upper syringe for womb, &c., with screw for various attachments; lower for hypodermic (under the skin) injections.

Remedy.—Siphon or syringe uterus with tepid water and antiseptic. Remove remnants of placenta (the afterbirth) or blood clots; treat any wounds antiseptically. Where walls of uterus are dilated or flaccid, inject solution of ergot and belladonna tincture. Rugs wrung out of hot water over loins and abdomen, relieve spasm and pain. Sulpho-carbolates, sulphites, or hydronaphthol internally. If bowels are torpid, half dose of physic, with ginger, gentian, and molasses, and promote effect by laxative injections. Remove urine by catheter. Sustain the strength by generous diet, tonics, and stimulants. Separate from pregnant or suckling animals. Disinfect.

HYSTERIA

Is usually caused by sexual heat. Sometimes it is the result of nervous, convulsive, or spasmodic affections. Breeding is perhaps the best remedy for sexual heat.

Symptoms.—Clenching jaws, grinding teeth, squinting; unrelaxing spasms alternated with relaxing; kicking, stamping, and other signs of nervous excitement; sometimes rapid opening and closing of vulva, &c.

INFLAMMATION OF THE TESTICLES.

Remedy.—Fomentations, anodynes, a dose of physic, support testicle. Iodine liniment; potassium iodide internally. Tubercular form intractable; castrate in early stage. For doses, see pages 13 to 29.

PROTRUDED PENIS (PARAPHYMOSIS),

Is sometimes caused by loss of power (paralysis). In the stallion there are many other causes, such as excessive copulation, friction before copulation, by rubbing against female; kicks and other injuries; introduction into anus; attempt to cover a 'ringed mare;' irritating substances (medicines) in prepuce; warts, &c.

Remedy.—Amputate if necessary.

Confined (unprotrudable) Penis (phymosis) is very rare.

Amputation of the Penis is practicable, and is sometimes resorted to as a cure for warts, ulcers, cancer, protrusion, &c.

Cancerous Tumor of the Vulva is recorded. As it did not yield to treatment, but gradually enlarged till it filled "two-thirds of the vulva," the mare was destroyed. The tumor existed nearly three years.

Dropsy of the Womb (Hydrometra), causes great distention of the belly. In a recorded case the uterus was filled with six quarts of thick, white matter, resembling healthy pus.

Diseases of the Ovaries usually consist of watery or bloody tumors, sometimes accompanied by dropsy. The tumors, which sometimes weigh as much as 30 lbs., may become cancerous.

Abscess of the Scrotum is described by Percivall. The swelling filled one side of the scrotum of a gelding. It was opened and then fomented. Cured.

Self-Abuse is not very rare in stallions. The remedy is a net made for the purpose.

DISEASES OF THE HEART.

DISEASES of the heart are best distinguished from pulmonary diseases, with which they are often confounded, by auscultation. The heart's beats may be felt, heard, and counted, in either health or disease, and can therefore be contrasted. The contrast between the action of a healthy and a diseased heart should be carefully studied. Apply the flat of the hand or the ear to the *left* side, just behind the elbow. The stethoscope (a hollow or perforated piece of wood) may also be used. In health two successive sounds, followed by an interval of silence, are heard. Exercise and agitation increase the heart's action.

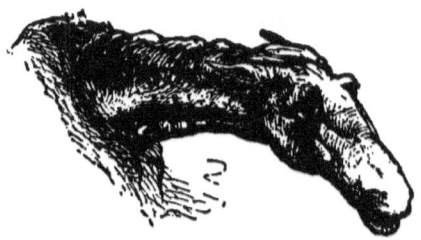

Fig. 27. A horse with Heart Disease.

Persistent coldness of the extremities, swelling of the legs, chest, and abdomen, fainting fits, dizziness, languor, difficult breathing, especially after severe exertion, are more or less constant symptoms of heart disease.

Disease of the heart is either the result of functional disturbance or structural alteration. Disease of the heart and its membranes may be either acute or chronic.

INFLAMMATION OF THE PERICARDIUM (PERICARDITIS).

The pericardium is the watery, membranous bag that contains the heart. Pericarditis may be the result of cold, exposure, or fatigue, but it is oftener the result of rheumatic fever, strangles, influenza, purpura, blood contaminations, diseases of the lungs, pleura, and heart itself, cancer, parasitic growths, wounds, &c.

The disease, says Percivall, usually follows or is secondary to pleurisy. The effusions of water and lymph peculiar to pleurisy are often found within the pericardium, "as though one membrane had sympathized with the other." The lymph is mostly disposed in layers on the internal surface of the sac and the exterior of the heart to such a degree as to cause adhesion between the two. It is of an albuminous character. In time, when lining the pericardium, it becomes firm, thin, and white. In a recorded case it was of the nature of cartilage, and about an eighth of an inch in thickness.

The symptoms of pericarditis are exceedingly variable. (Robertson.)

Remedy.—Cautious bleeding, followed by small doses of aconite, is serviceable in acute independent cases, but is unsuitable in second stages or in epizootic attacks.

Morphine hypodermically usually relieves acute pain. Woolen cloths wrung out of hot water to chest for an hour or two at a time. Soap liniment, 1-20th part opium tincture, rubbed in freely between fomentations. Sodium bicarbonate and sulphate in drinking water relieve fever and maintain action of bowels. Digitalis may be used carefully when heart action is feeble and rapid. In more advanced stage, and when fluid is effused, supporting treatment needful. Moderate doses of stimulants; potassium or ferrous iodide, with mustard or cantharides to chest. Digitalis and strychnine assist absorption of fluid by raising blood pressure in kidney arteries and promoting urination.

Where dropsy of the pericardium (hydrops pericardi), persists, remove fluid by special trocar. This is sometimes described as a distinct disease.

For doses, see pages 13 to 29.

PALPITATION OF THE HEART

Is usually tumultuous and rapid action. Sometimes there is a peculiar sound and irregular heart and arterial pulsations. Sometimes the heart action seems completely confused, and sometimes there is intermittency. The palpitation may be continuous or only at intervals.

The causes of palpitation may be too much blood, blood contamination, poverty of blood, &c. Nervous and excitable temperament, debility, exhaustion, and youth are said to be predisposing causes.

Remedy.—Rest, quiet, generous diet. Iron tonics for anæmic murmurs (a sound caused by deficiency of blood). Small doses of aconite for violent action. Digitalis for weak and irregular action. Bromides for irregular and fluttering action. Laxatives for digestive derangement. Belladonna for strain or overexertion. Strychnine is a heart tonic. (For a list of heart and other tonics, see page 37.)

Where there is fainting or loss of sensation and motion, dash cold water over the head; ammonia to nostrils. If the condition results from loss of blood, transfuse blood from a healthy and vigorous horse.

For doses, see pages 13 to 29.

OTHER HEART DISEASES.

There are other heart diseases, such as inflammation of both the membrane and substance of the heart (endocarditis and carditis); both enlargement and wasting of the heart; fatty changes in the heart; rupture of the heart, and also the pericardium; adventitious growths in connection with the heart, such as parasitic and malignant, fibroid and vascular tumors; disease of the valves and orifices; ossification (rare); air in the heart; enlargement of the aorta.

The symptoms of most of these affections — many of which are rare — are puzzling even to veterinarians.

Where heart disease is suspected, avoid overwork and excitement.

DISEASES OF THE LIVER.

DISEASES of the liver are somewhat rare in horses. The probable cause is simplicity of diet. Hot climates, as in man, seem to be conducive of equine liver disease. Liver diseases are often insidious. They are sometimes mistaken for lung diseases. Next to the lungs the liver seems to be the most frequent seat of tubercles. Sometimes it is soft or rotten and clay colored; sometimes hard and tough, the color, however, being natural.

INFLAMMATION OF THE LIVER (HEPATITIS),

Seems to be of three kinds or degrees—the cover or membrane, the substance of the liver, or both. Percivall and Williams give the following

Symptoms.—Dull; head heavy; eyes drooping and lusterless; occasional cough; no appetite; apparent inward pain, but not acute; stands up; very feverish; in two or three days the fever or diffused bile causes the mouth and eyes to become yellow, the blood golden-hued and specked with yellow, floating particles; dung balls imbued with bile and sometimes coated with viscid, bilious, mucous-like, reddish-brown matter, leaving an opium-like stain when rubbed on white paper; urine scanty and thick, with bilious tinge and copious sediment; may lie on left side, but soon rises; right side tender, if not somewhat swollen; when standing, points (rests) the off (right) fore limb; pulse quick, strong, bounding; breathing sometimes disturbed, sometimes not; stupid; dizzy; staggers; danger of apoplexy or bursting of liver.

DISEASES OF THE LIVER.

Remedy.—Purgatives, salines, ammonia chloride. Aconite for fever. Ipecac. Foment and stimulate over liver. Digestible, laxative food. Exercise after relief of acute symptoms. Nitro-hydrochloric acid in chronic cases. Salines and careful dietary safer than more active remedies when the inflammation or congestion is associated with epizootic or other disease. For doses, see pages 13 to 29.

Congestion of the Liver.—Robertson describes three kinds—the passive, the active, and the biliary. These, which may be the result of lung or heart disease, sudden chills, specific fevers, blood contamination, too much or improper food, lack of exercise, &c., seem to be preludes to inflammation of the liver.

Robertson also describes 'Scirrhosis of the Liver,' a chronic or subacute inflammation of the interconnective liver tissue; 'Fatty Liver,' 'Albuminoid or Lardaceous (lard or wax) Liver,' &c.

Liver Concretions.—Rigot found 90 concretions in the bile ducts of a liver. The cavities were enlarged and their walls thickened, but there were no indications of liver disease during life. The same horse had a salivary calculus (stone).

Hydatid Tumors of the Liver are rare. They are bladder-like, and vary in size from a hazel-nut to an orange, containing a clear fluid and numerous organisms (mites). They cause very little if any disturbance.

Rupture of the Liver is caused by external violence, overdistention with blood or bile, &c. Fatal.

JAUNDICE OR YELLOWS (ICTERUS).

Is a symptom of disease rather than disease itself. It is usually attributed to either deranged bile secretion or bile distribution. When the bile is taken into the blood instead of its natural channel—the alimentary canal—it imparts a yellow tinge to the eyes, nose, mouth, skin, urine, and sometimes the dung. The latter is sometimes clay colored. Sometimes the bowels are deranged and there is a "defective movement of the right fore limb," a dry, scurfy, and itchy state of the skin, loss of appetite, strength, &c.

Remedy.—In ordinary cases light, digestible food will sometimes suffice. A laxative, alternated with salines, clears away excess of bile, and promotes a healthy action of the liver. Ammonia chloride and salines useful where a case is complicated with duodenal catarrh. (The duodenum is the first of the small intestines.)

When depending on suppression of bile, apply mustard or other stimulant over liver. Thickened ox bile, in bolus, twice a day, with moderate doses of aromatic spirit of ammonia between. Nitro-hydrochloric acid, and quinine with it when the patient is weak.

For doses, see pages 13 to 29.

Little relief can be given in jaundice when it is caused by scirrhosis or fatty degeneration.

DISEASES OF THE SPLEEN.

Diseases of the spleen are somewhat rare, but some of them, such as moderate enlargement, &c., may exist for years without causing serious inconvenience. The spleen weighs from 3 to 4 pounds. When enlarged it sometimes weighs from 14 to 20 and even 50 pounds.

Percivall describes inflammation, cancer, and rupture of the spleen. Williams says atrophy (wasting), thrombosis (coagulation of blood), tubercle, cancer, hydatids, and ossification are found after death. He also says that American horses suffer from an intermittent fever in which the spleen becomes enlarged. Robertson describes surface growths of the spleen, the same in size as those of the liver (from hazel-nut to orange), of grayish-white color and usually firm consistence, with an immense number of tubercle-bacilli (mites). Some of these latter cases cause much debility.

DISEASES OF THE EYES.

PERIODIC OPHTHALMIA (MOON-BLINDNESS),

Is a specific inflammation of most of the structures of the eye. Relapses occur, lasting from 2 to 14 days. It is dangerous, and is liable to be followed by a still more dangerous disease—cataract. It is hereditary, but it may be caused by rheumatic predisposition or blood contamination, a bite or blow, foreign substances under the lid, overwork, especially the young, filthy and badly ventilated stables, the eruption of the tushes, compression of the roots of the molar teeth on the fifth pair of nerves, working in coal-pits or other dark places, &c.

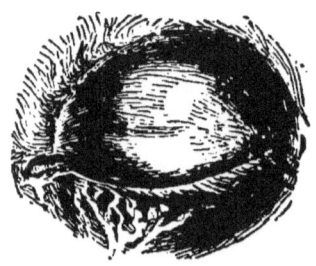

Fig. 28. First appearance of Periodic Ophthalmia.

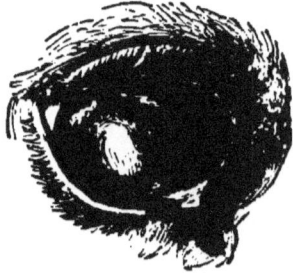

Fig. 29. Its termination.

Symptoms.—First or inflammatory stage: Upper lid droops; tears in superabundance; lids, venous vessels, and conjunctive membrane swollen; the globe dull and sunken; circumference of cornea sometimes exhibits a broad, nebulous circle; front chamber, at first usually clear, becomes so obscured that the pupil is hardly distinguishable; the pupil is contracted and resembles the black eye of a garden bean; cornea, if not already, soon becomes obscured; this obscures the pupil and iris.

Second stage: Gradual decline of inflammation and tardy clearing of the cornea; iris altered in color and lusterless; pupil contracted but less sensitive to light; whitish or yellowish lymph effusions in chamber; these and other favorable signs indicate recovery, but a relapse usually occurs in a few days.

Remedy.—The periodic or specific form is incurable, but it is relieved by purges, febrifuges, anodynes, belladonna, or atrophine locally and internally.

For simple inflammation of the eye, occurring in all

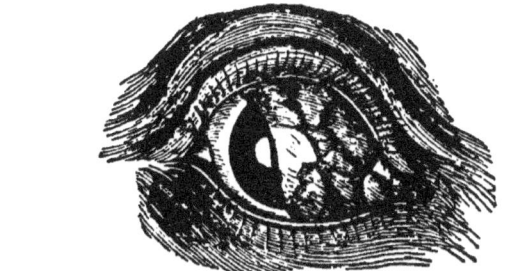

Fig. 30. The haw.

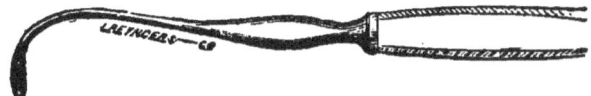

Fig. 31. Tenaculum.

animals: Remove any foreign body, securing the haw, if necessary, with a tenaculum or stitch. Fomentation with tepid water and decoction of poppy-heads abates irritation, whether depending on foreign body or cold. Half dose physic. Where inflammation severe, bleed from angular vein. Belladonna and atrophine, locally and generally, diminish irritation and prevent adhesion of iris. Steam head when occurring with swelled lids, as in influenza attacks. Shade the eye.

Silver nitrate and other astringent solutions for chronic cases. For doses, see pages 13 to 29.

CATARACT

Is opacity of the lens or its capsule. Percivall says it may also be the result of an effusion of an opaque fluid between the two. The opacity may be the result of injury or disease.

Cataract is a common cause of either total or partial blindness. It usually follows ophthalmia, but ophthalmia may attack a cataractous eye. Cataracts are white, black, green, yellow, brown, ash-colored, &c. At first they are soft, but they acquire firmness by age. Some are called

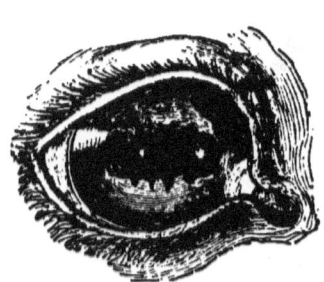

Fig. 32. Partial Cataract.

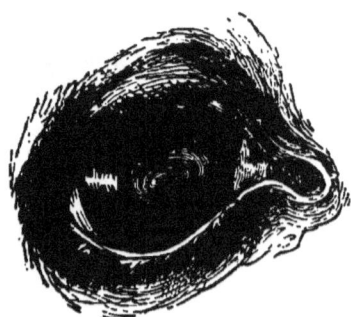

Fig. 33. Complete Cataract.

bony cataracts. They vary in size from a pin's point to a pea.

Percivall speaks of both spontaneous and congenital cataracts; D'Arboval of a fluid cataract, which, from its whiteness, is called milky; Gibson of colts being foaled with cataracts or pearls in their eyes.

Lenticular cataracts grow slowly—1, 2, or more years. The other kinds may appear in a few days, or even hours, and without any detectible inflammation or previous disease. Capsular cataract is caused usually perhaps by external injury. It is easily distinguished, and seems to be absorbable.

In cataract with ophthalmia the iris frequently becomes contracted and adheres to the capsule of the lens, thus causing a permanently small pupil.

Remedy.—Extraction by operation. Belladonna or atrophine dilate the pupil for diagnosis (distinguishment), alternated with physostygmine for obtaining free movement of iris. Phosphoreted oil, instilled into human eye, if borne, leads to final absorption.

For doses, see pages 13 to 29.

Green Cataract (Glaucoma), is opacity of the vitreous humor (glass-like fluid) of the eye. Incurable. Cutting out (iridectomy) affords relief. Physostygmine diminishes intraocular pressure (pressure within the eye).

AMAUROSIS OR GUTTA SERENA (GLASS-EYE),

Is caused by paralysis of the optic nerve and retina. There may be many causes of the paralysis, such as diseases of remote as well as contiguous parts, excessive bleeding, narcotic poisons, drinking too much cold water when heated, pressure from a tumor, &c. There is no visible defect in the eye—nothing abnormal except its great brilliancy, from which it takes its name.

Symptoms.—Head and ears erect, the latter set in motion to learn the cause of any alarming noise; lofty step; eyes insensible to light; pupils usually fixed and widely dilated; sometimes there is a sluggish motion and only moderate dilatation, &c.

Remedy.—Except when depending on brain disorder or debility, it is incurable. Blisters; setons around orbit. Strychnine in traumatic (wound) cases; also those of nerve wasting, but unsuitable where there are brain symptoms. For doses, see pages 13 to 29.

WORM IN THE EYE

Is rare in this country, but is common in India. It is like "an eel in a basin of water," but is not always in sight, for it may hide behind the iris. Dr. Gibbs (of India) has seen two worms in an eye at once. He has also seen a second worm appear months after the removal of the first. They are peculiar to cold weather and wet seasons. Similar worms are found in the stomach and intestines. They probably reach the eyes through the blood. If no operation is performed, blindness may result. But the worm may die and become absorbed.

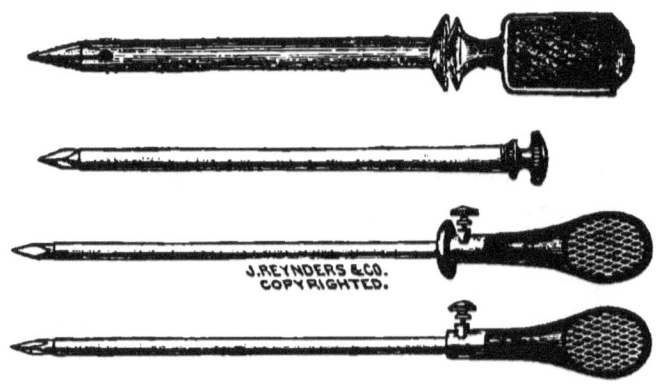

Fig. 34. Trocars. An operation for Worm in the Eye would require a special trocar.

The only remedy of course is to trocar or lance the eye, an operation the skillful surgeon only can perform.

"WATERY EYES"

Are uncommon. The real cause of the overflow of tears is obstruction of the tear canals, which run from the eyes to the nostrils; but superabundant secretion of tears may sometimes occur perhaps. It seems to be analogous to stricture of the urethra in man. The canal is not uniform in size, diminishing at first, then enlarging, besides which it is tortuous near its center.

Remedy.—Syringe from above, and below also, if necessary. If this fails, probe.

ENLARGEMENT OF THE LACHRYMAL CARUNCLE.

The lachrymal caruncle is a small, reddish, follicular body, situate at the inner angle of the eye. It is harmless when small. Its removal is sometimes followed by more or less inflammation and sometimes "watery eyes." Percivall removed one as large as a marble by ligature, tightening the cord on the second, fourth, and sixth days, when the excrescence (for such it had become) fell off. The operation caused great local disturbance, but it did not show itself till twelve days afterward. Bathing the eye, purging, and salivation with calomel followed. Recovered.

TUMORS AND FUNGUS OF THE ORBIT.

Percivall operated successfully on an exostosis (bony tumor) of the orbital arch, which had grown to the size of a horse-chestnut. It half eclipsed and pressed upon the eye. Doctor Perry treated a 3-days-old foal that was said "to have no eyes." He found a fungus within the orbit of the near side about the size of a pistol-ball, without any organic structure. That of the other orbit was of similar appearance, but somewhat larger, with the addition of the haw.

All tumors interfering with the sight or the movements of the eye should be removed.

DISEASES OF THE TEETH, MOUTH, LIPS, ETC.

DECAY OR CARIES OF THE TEETH

Is rare, especially in young horses. The back teeth or molars suffer more than the front teeth (incisors). They are sometimes broken by stones or other hard substances in the food. A severe blow over their roots sometimes causes caries and the ultimate loss of the tooth. It is possible to stop decay, especially of the front teeth, by filling.

Care of the teeth is a matter of great importance. Mastication of the food is indispensable to digestion, and digestion to health. Owing to the fact that horses' teeth (except the tushes, which are practically useless), grow throughout life—the growth counteracting the wear and the wear the growth—sharp and dangerous projections sometimes cause lacerations. When the teeth meet in perfect apposition—grinding surface to grinding surface—the wear is regular; when they do not, the unworn parts will soon project. When they cause laceration of the cheek or tongue, file them, but do not interfere with the natural slant of the tables (crown or grinding surfaces). The natural slant must be preserved, or mastication cannot be properly performed. The molar teeth of the horse are in this respect the reverse of human teeth.

Supernumerary teeth and dental cysts require surgical skill. The so-called wolf teeth (really remnant teeth, for they are the remains of what were once functionally developed teeth), that appear in front of the first upper molars, sometimes cause more or less trouble. It is better to extract them, which any one can do with ordinary forceps.

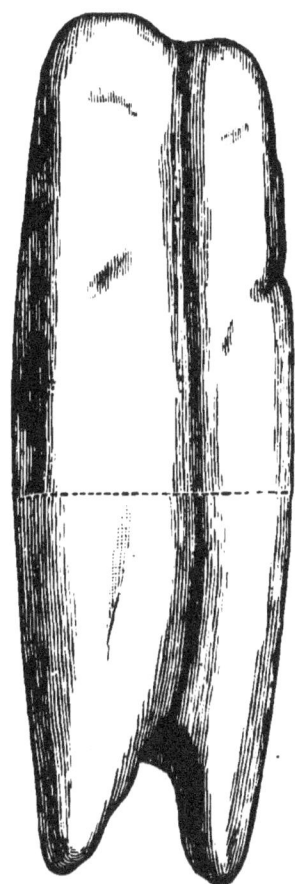

Fig. 35. Abnormal growth begins at dotted line.

Figure 35 represents a back molar tooth which, on account of the loss of the opposite tooth, grew till it killed the horse.

PARROT-MOUTH

Consists in the upper front teeth—from irregularity and overgrowth—projecting in front of the lower, like the upper bill of the parrot. The lower incisors are liable, also from overgrowth, to injure the roof of the mouth. Grazing is difficult and sometimes almost impracticable; but the animal may be fed from the manger. The remedy is usually only palliative. Forceps, files, and surgical

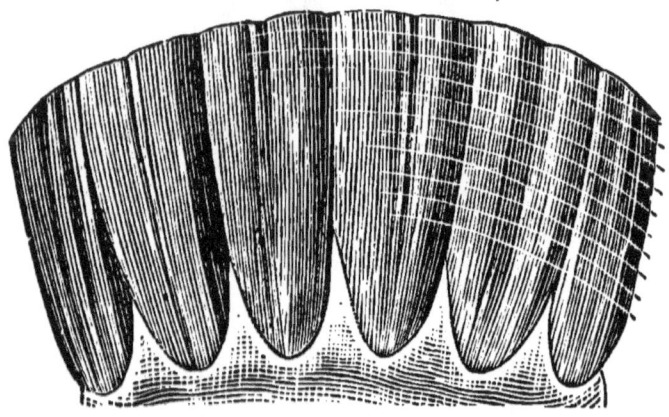

Fig. 36. Parrot-Mouth; teeth grown ten lines too long.

skill are required, not only for parrot-mouth, but for many other irregularities of the teeth, molars as well as incisors.

CRIB-BITING

Is doubly injurious to the horse. It wears and sometimes breaks its teeth and gives it the colic—crib-biters' colic—which is caused by the sucking in of air. Further, loss of saliva impairs digestion. The vice is a species of unsoundness. Breaking the front teeth interferes with grazing.

Remedy.—Iron stable fittings. Manger, when not in use, turned into recess in wall. Use muzzle or spiked neck-strap. Concentrated, digestible food. Chalk, antacids, and an occasional laxative relieve the indigestion from which crib-biters usually suffer. Separate crib-biters from other horses, as they imitate and acquire the habit. For a list of antacids, see page 31.

DENTAL INSTRUMENTS.

PLATE I.

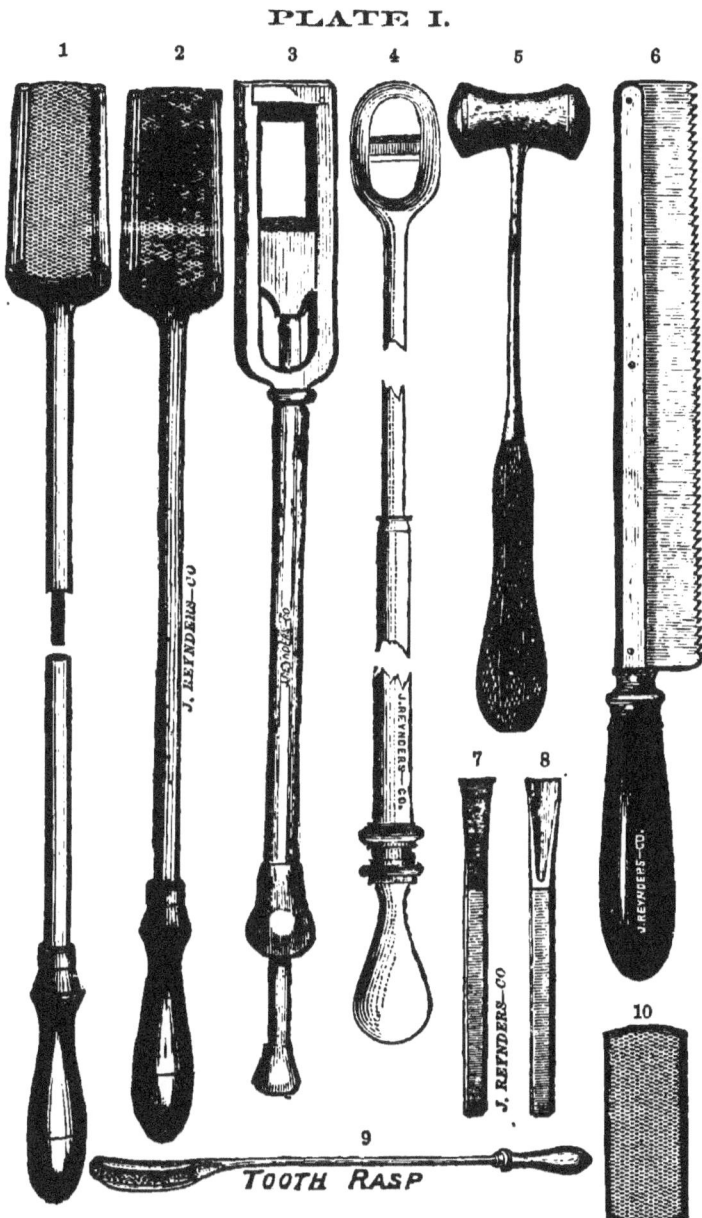

DENTAL INSTRUMENTS. 147

PLATE II.

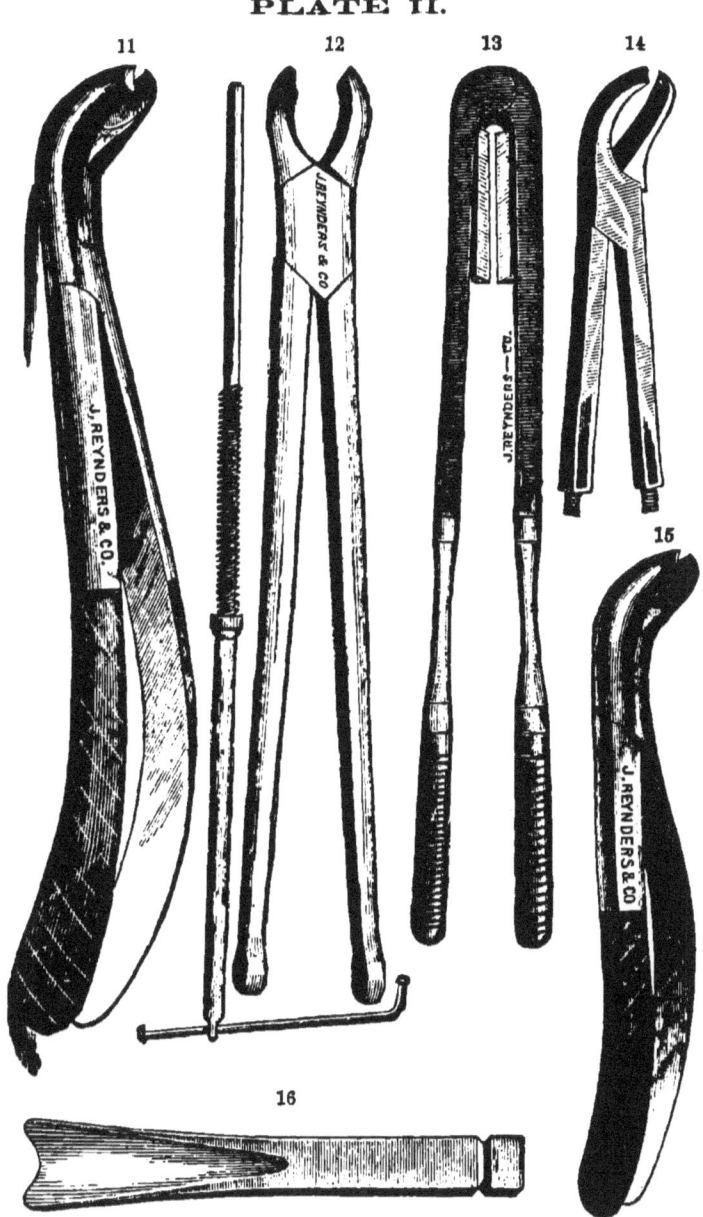

DENTAL INSTRUMENTS.

PLATE III.

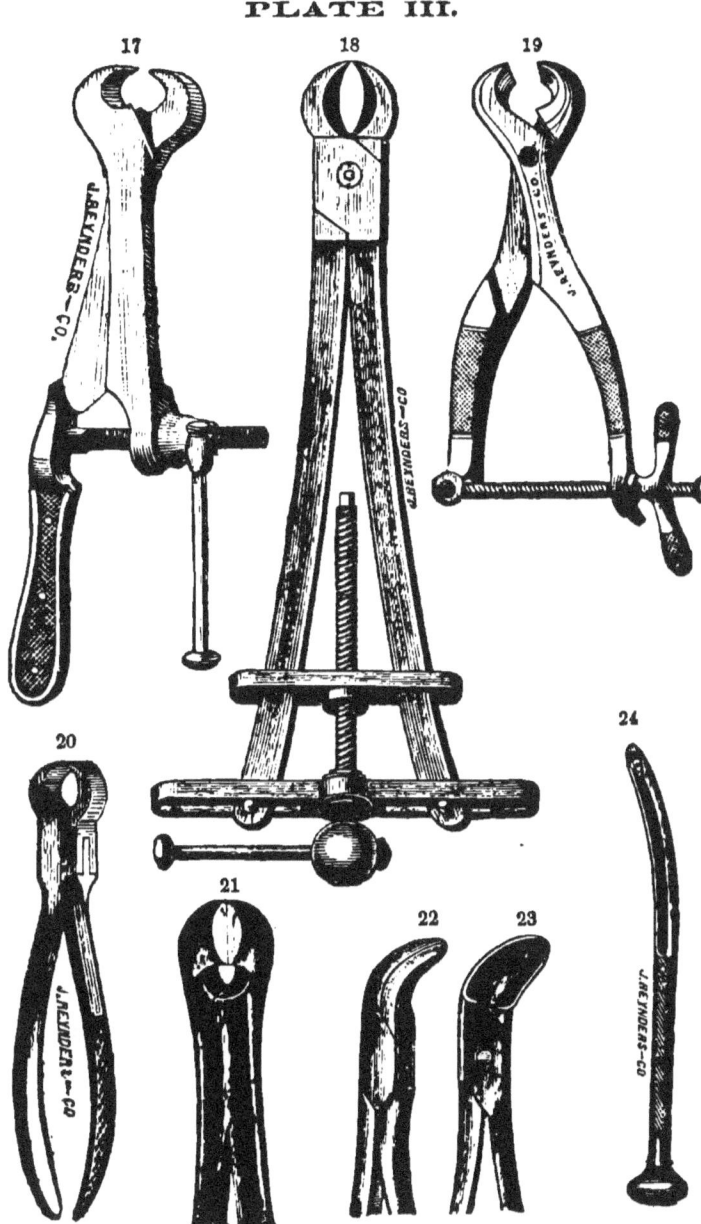

DENTAL INSTRUMENTS. 151

PLATE IV.

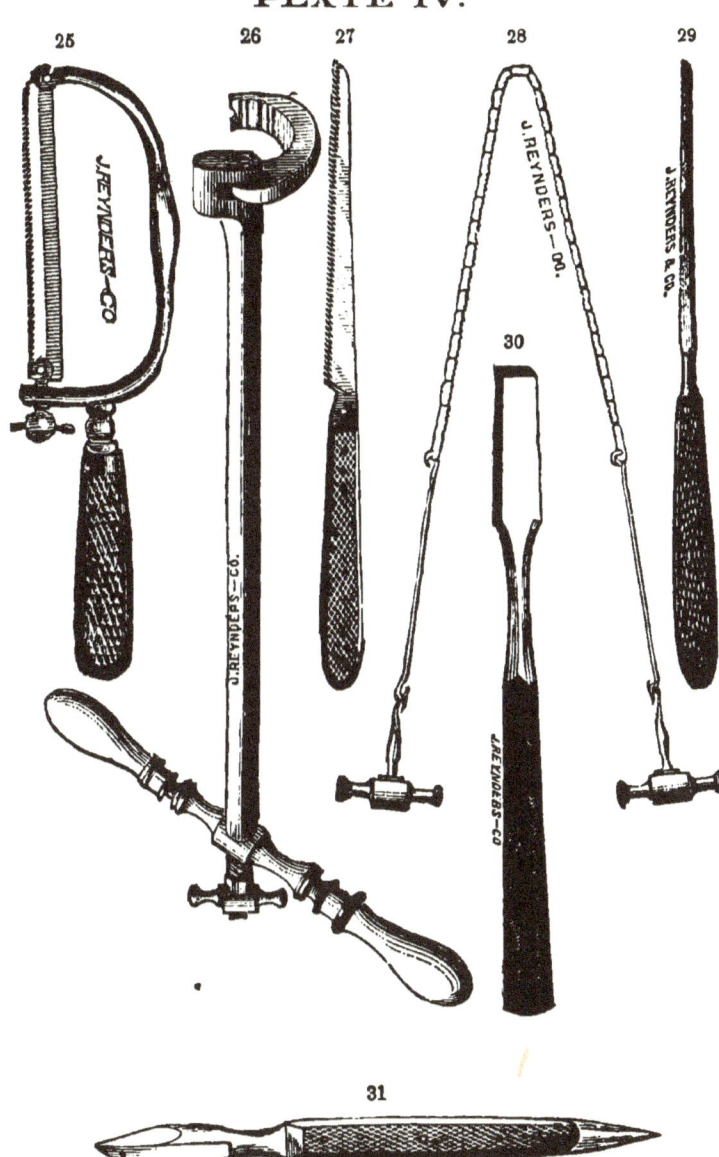

NAMES OF THE INSTRUMENTS.

1, 2, Adjustable Tooth Files. 3, Going's Tooth Chisel. 4, French model of same. 5, Tooth Mallet. 6, French model Tooth Saw. 7, Narrow Tooth Chisel. 8, Narrow Tooth Gouge. 9, Tooth Rasp, guarded. 10, Extra blade for Adjustable File. 11, Heavy Forceps. 12, Going's Forceps. 13, House's Cutting Forceps. 14, House's Pulling Forceps. 15, Wolf Tooth Forceps. 16, Wide Chisel. 17, Cutting Forceps, French model. 18, Moller's Cutting Forceps. 19, Cutting Forceps, French model. 20, 21, 22, 23, House's Cutting Forceps. 24, Narrow Gouge. 25, Bow Tooth Saw. 26, Key. 27. Plain Tooth Saw. 28, Chain Tooth Saw. 29, Fine ferruled Tooth Saw. 30, Narrow Tooth Chisel. 31, Hurlburt's Gum Knife and Tooth Pick.

LAMPAS

Is congestion, fever and swelling of the gums and bars of the mouth. It is peculiar to the young, but occurs sometimes in the aged also. The eruption of the teeth, especially the tushes, is probably the chief cause in the case of the young, and their continuous growth throughout life the chief cause in that of the old. Direct irritation, bits, the action of certain foods, and gastric disorder are also causes.

The remedy is lancing the gums and bars. Let the blood out. Burning is not only useless but barbarous. Soft or green food and astringent wash if necessary.

INFLAMMATION OF THE MOUTH (STOMATITIS),

Is simple or catarrhal, vesicular, pustular, and ulcerative. It is peculiar to the young, and is attributed to defective sanitary conditions, improper diet, and the effect of wasting diseases.

A contagious pustular form of the disease occurred in Berlin, Prussia, in 1876.

Remedy.—Careful feeding, laxatives, salines for gastric disorder. In sucking foals and calves, besides local treatment, see that the mother's milk is healthy and that she is properly fed. Potassium chlorate or borax and glycerine solution. Dress ulcers with glycerite of tannin, or paint with silver nitrate, 10 grains to ounce of water.

For doses, see pages 13 to 29.

INFLAMMATION OF THE TONGUE (GLOSSITIS),

Is rare.

Remedy.—Irrigate with mild astringent solutions. Apply bismuth, oxymel, molasses, or vinegar. Soft, nutritive food. Scarify if the swelling is extensive. If laxatives cannot be given per mouth, inject. For doses, see pages 13 to 29.

Tumor of the Lip, usually the lower, causes more or less swelling. It is about the size of a pigeon's egg, has a firm feel, is hot, and gives pain when pressed. Its origin may, as a rule, be spontaneous, but it has been known to arise from a bite or a sting. It usually bursts internally in two or three days, discharging pus. Cleanse and inject with a solution of alum or borax daily.

Tumor of the Face is peculiar to young horses and usually appears on the side, between the eye and the angle of the mouth. Like other exostoses, they grow from the bone; are round, broad at their bases, with little heat and very little tenderness. They may be caused by blows, and perhaps also by caries (bone rot). They do no great harm unless they become fistulous; but they greatly disfigure the face.

Salivary Calculi (stone-like concretions), are sometimes found in the salivary glands, usually within their canals, the parotid duct (canal), &c. An oat or other substance penetrates the canal, or possibly pierces the cheek. It is the nucleus for a stone-like or tartar-like concretion. Its growth is slow. Sometimes it is superficial in depth, when it can be seen or felt; but sometimes it is deep. Sometimes it lacerates the membrane of the mouth, grating against the teeth. It will usually more or less obstruct the flow of saliva. Sometimes it causes swelling.

Stricture of the Esophagus (Œsophagus) is rare and usually fatal. The tube (throat) sometimes becomes so contracted at the part affected that it will not admit the little finger. As the horse cannot swallow solid food, death results from starvation.

Dr. Cheetham treated a case successfully by opening

the tube and passing probangs. The first, an inch and a half in diameter, was followed by larger ones, which were passed two or three times a day for ten days. Afterward the owner of the animal passed the probang occasionally himself. The stricture was seated at the point where the tube enters the chest. A sac or pouch three or four inches in diameter had formed near the stricture, and had acted as a receptacle for food.

Rupture of the Esophagus.—Dr. Cartwright reports a case of rupture eight inches long that "had evidently been made with some sharp or rough instrument." The mare died in eight days. A sheep's probang stopped at one-third of the neck.

Opening the Esophagus.—The esophagus lies near but is deeper than, and, toward its center, somewhat to the left of the windpipe. The incision must be made carefully on account of the proximity of the jugular veins, carotid arteries, &c. If the nature of the case will permit, open the left side of the neck, three inches longitudinally below its upper third, or near or at its center. An assistant should press on the jugular. Near the windpipe will be found "a firm, cordiform, shining, red substance." This is the esophagus. Draw it outward with a blunt hook, and make a longitudinal incision. Use a tube if the case requires it. When through, stitch the esophagus with silk and close the external wound with pins. Apply a compress. Give liquid or soft food till the wound heals.

Choking is usually the result of improper mastication and greediness. Whole grains of corn, a small potato, large pieces of turnip, egg shells, a hard ball of food— even of grass—will sometimes lodge in the throat. Sometimes a draft of water or the hand will clear the passage, but a probang is usually necessary. A cane, flexible if to be had, a whalebone, the butt end of a whip, or any similar instrument will answer the purpose.

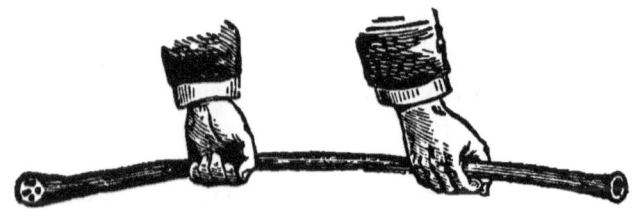

Fig. 37. The Probang.

Dr. Holmes saved a horse from choking by opening the esophagus and removing the obstruction. Dr. King saved another by cutting down to the esophagus only. Finding the obstruction, a ball of medicine, pliable, he manipulated it. It was then washed down with water.

DISEASES OF THE SKIN.

DISEASES of the skin, though common, are of less importance relatively than many other diseases; but they are deserving of careful attention notwithstanding this fact. Inability to perform work, not to mention disfigurement, alone renders the subject worthy of study. It is noteworthy that a remedy that benefits one skin disease will benefit others more or less. The diseases may be caused by agencies from without as well as from within, both of which must be considered in the treatment.

Two liniments suitable for persistent skin diseases, enlarged glands, and chronic indurations (hardened parts) are as follows:

1. Mercurial ointment, 2 ounces; camphor, 1 dram; oil of tar, 3 ounces; linseed oil, 4 ounces.

2. Mercurial ointment, 2 ounces; creosote, 1 dram; liquor ammoniæ, 2 ounces; linseed oil, 6 ounces.

ERYTHEMA (Red, Rose-Colored),

Is a superficial inflammation of the skin, usually occurring in patches more or less extensive, with sometimes a certain amount of effusion into the deeper layers. It is non-contagious, independent or symptomatic, active or passive.

There are several forms of the disease—among them mud fever—the mildest of which are troublesome. It often results from injury. The patches are slightly elevated, sometimes with well-defined margins, at others gradually shading off into the healthy skin. There is more or less exudation, scaling, and itching.

Remedy.—Laxatives, especially in gastro-intestinal irritation. Salines in drinking water, such as Epsom salt. Bicarbonate of potash and glycerine, or glycerine and water. When the chafing is severe, a solution of tannic acid with glycerine; or an ointment of tannic acid and opium; or paint with a weak solution of nitrate of silver 1 part to 12 of water; or dust with flour. Blisters, diuretics, and arsenic and quinine internally if necessary.

For doses, see pages 13 to 29.

Horses liable to mud fever should not have the hair of the leg removed, nor should the legs be washed.

NETTLE-RASH OR SURFEIT (URTICARIA),

Consists of irregularly distributed patches of nettle-sting-like eruptions; soft, but possessing moderate resistance to the touch. The patches usually appear and disappear with

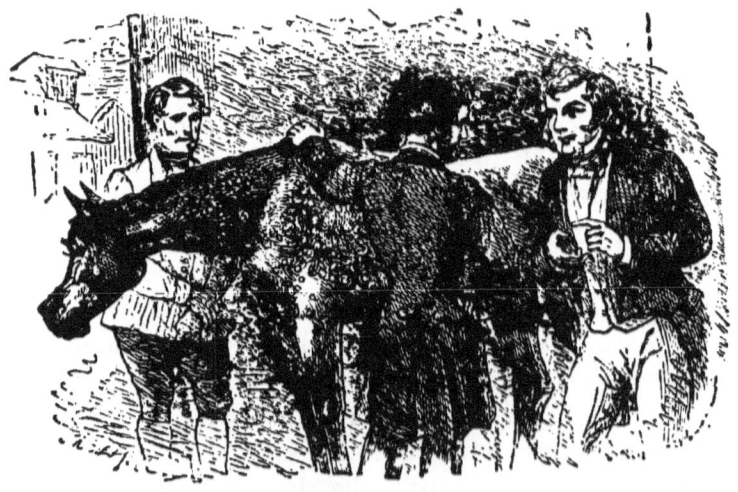

Fig. 38. Nettle-Rash or Surfeit.

equal rapidity, sometimes in a few hours. In some cases, however, they persist for a week. One crop may follow another. There is little scaling, but more or less itching. Sometimes the coat remains slightly open for a while.

The horse is often languid and moderately feverish. In a few cases the bowels and kidneys are affected. When the patches appear around the eyes and throat they disfigure the horse and threaten serious results.

The disease usually appears in the spring, and is usually caused by high feeding and little work. Percivall says the eruptions may attack the air passages.

Remedy.—Wash: Bichloride of mercury, 12 grains; dilute hydrocyanic acid, 4 drams; glycerine or almond mixture, 2 ounces; water, 10 ounces. A laxative and attention to diet. Salines, antiseptics, and tonics are serviceable in debilitated subjects.

For doses, see pages 13 to 29.

LICHEN (Pimples) AND PRURIGO (Itching),

Are described by Robertson as different forms of skin papulation (pimples). Both are chronic rather than acute. In lichen the pimples are relatively larger in the horse than in man. By abrasion there may be much exudation and crusting in both lichen and prurigo. In lichen the pimples do not suppurate, but they shed bran-like scales. In prurigo they are more varied in size and are further apart. The skin is hard, dry, and wrinkled. There are collections of pus beneath the crusts, great shedding of scales, itching, and sometimes swelling of the lymphatic glands, with constitutional disturbance. Parasites are sometimes present.

The causes of these diseases seem to be more general or constitutional than local. Malassimilation and defective nutrition seem to be important factors. Heredity is probable.

Remedy.—If the animal is weak, good food, fresh air, tonics. If strong, gentle purge, moderate but daily doses of salines, such as sulphate of soda or magnesia. For severe itching 2 or 3 applications of the following mixture: Nitrate of silver, 2 grains; cyanide of potassium, 3 grains; water 1 ounce. Sulphur iodide and wood tar oils are alternated night and morning when the skin in chronic cases is much thickened.

For doses, see pages 13 to 29.

ECZEMA (CUTANEOUS CATARRH),

Of which there are four varieties, seems to be an inflammation of the superficial layers of the skin, accompanied by pimples, vesicles, or pustules, itching, and sometimes scales and partial baldness. It is one of the commonest skin diseases, and is liable to be confounded with other diseases of its class, especially itch and erysipelas. It is exudative or moist, and is caused apparently by anything that disturbs the healthy action of the skin. It is the result sometimes perhaps of nerve paralysis. It is disposed to appear in successive crops, and is usually independent. It is most frequent over the neck, trunk, quarters and around some of the orifices. The eruptive discharges, sometimes sero-purulent, are disposed to collect in crusts, which, if rubbed, aggravate and prolong the disease.

Remedy.—Simple form: Laxative, cooling diet. Prevent biting and rubbing. Clip long hair. As vesicles dry, apply zinc oxide and kaolin, alternated with tar oil. Where discharges are profuse and skin puffy, apply astringents dry; zinc oxide, mixed with 6 or 8 parts kaolin or starch, or dust surfaces with bismuth ternitrate.

More inflammatory and moist form: Cleanse with soap and water. Soak repeatedly with mercurous oxide wash, and dress with zinc oxide ointment. Lead acetate with glycerine and water for the inflammatory weeping stages. Stronger lead lotions, with chloroform or laudanum, or both, for dry, itching surfaces. Where spots are limited, paint with 2 grains silver nitrate to ounce of water, or water and glycerine. Laxatives, salines, cooling diet for hot skin and fever.

Pus form: Mercurous oxide wash. Zinc or lead acetate solutions, watery or oleaginous. Occasional dressing with eucalyptol or thymol abate suppuration and itching. Opium and belladonna tinctures with astringents for irritation and pain. Attend to bowels and kidneys. Mineral acids and tonics internally. Digestible, nutritive diet.

Scales form: Soak crusts with oil till loose; remove. Stimulate skin with a dressing of 1 part oleum picis; 4 parts potassium carbonate and sublimed sulphur, and 30 each of lard and olive oil. Leave on 2 or 3 days. Wash off with soap and warm water. Wood tar oil or sulphur iodide locally. Continue acid and tonic treatment, and give arsenic. Hydrocyanic acid, potassium cyanide, benzoin, chloral, chloroform, camphor, or cocaine relieve the itching in all stages. A blister sometimes reëstablishes healthy action in chronic cases.

For doses, see pages 13 to 29.

Sublimed sulphur (flowers of sulphur) is prepared by distilling the crude sulphur and conducting it in the state of vapor into large chambers, where it condenses in a fine, spherically granulated, yellow powder.

HERPES (Creeping, Spreading),

Is usually of two kinds. The first, peculiar to sucking foals, is composed of vesicles somewhat larger than those of eczema, and is found in irregular patches at the junction of the skin with mucous membranes. The second, peculiar to adult life, is composed of pimples, vesicles, or pustules irregularly distributed over the body in circular patches, the hair of which soon falls off, exposing the eruptions and a slightly scaly skin. There is probably a parasitic form.

The eruptions do not often break, their contents being either absorbed or dried. For the first week they are disposed to spread, the hair around the margins appearing to die for want of nutrition, but reappearing when the scaling process is completed, usually in two or three weeks. There is little itching and rarely any noticeable constitutional disturbance. The disease is thought to be caused by nerve paralysis. It is probably not contagious.

Remedy.—Alkaline wash, after which rub in vaselin. Boro-glycerine with a drop of hydrocyanic acid for itching. Half doses of physic or salines remove the gastric derangement on which most cases depend. In foals see to the health of the mother and state of milk.

The spreading variety, persisting often for weeks, prob-

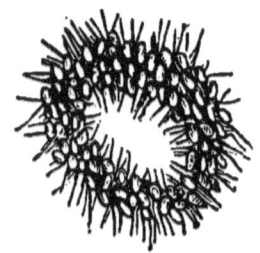

Fig. 39. Vesicles forming.

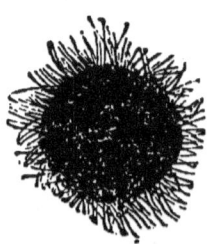

Fig. 40. Appearance after Vesicles have burst or evaporated.

ably caused by a parasite, is treated by dilute solution of iodine or other antiseptic. Pustular variety treated by half doses of physic, dressed with zinc oxide or boric acid. Itching abated by menthol. Growth of hair promoted by mild cantharides or other stimulant.

For doses, see pages 13 to 29.

ECTHYMA (Boil-Like Eruptions),

Is peculiar to American horses. It affects the deep layers of the skin, appearing mostly over the back and quarters where the harness rubs. The pustules, which have firm but much inflamed bases, mature in about a week, are moderately large, round, distinct, separate, and have well-marked points. The disease, which differs from true boil in that it does not have a core, is distinctively pustular, but some of the eruptions may at first discharge

SKIN DISEASES.

a straw-colored, sticky fluid. Most of the pustules emerge the first week; a few come later. They have dark-colored, somewhat persistent scabs, and when healed leave a temporarily indented scar.

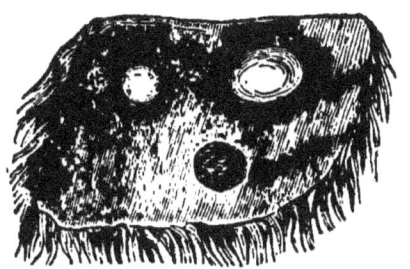

Fig. 41. Ecthyma.

The disease is probably caused by disturbed nutrition and particular as well as general debility. The parasites sometimes found in the running pustules are probably accidental deposits from the air.

Remedy.—Laxative salines relieve gastro-intestinal or other irritants. Exercise further hastens the removal of waste products. Digestible, rather laxative diet. A mild dose of aloes may be followed by 2 or 3 drams of sulphate of soda or magnesia, 2 or 3 times a day in drinking water; also, with the salines or separately, 2 to 4 fluid drams of dilute sulphuric acid.

Mineral acids, iron salts, bitters, arsenic, act as antiseptics and alteratives. Pustules treated by water dressing, boric acid, zinc oxide ointment. Isolate and disinfect, as the disease is sometimes contagious.

For doses, see pages 13 to 29.

PSORIASIS (Scaly Inflammation),

Has two forms, the local and the general. The latter is distinct, and is usually associated with considerable constitutional disturbance. Both forms, in fact, are so distinct that they are not likely to be mistaken for others.

Although purely a skin disease, horses of sluggish habits and lymphatic temperaments are more liable to it than others, and it may be hereditary. It occurs chiefly about the flexures or joints, especially the carpal and tarsal, causing lameness, mallenders of the fore leg and sallenders of the hind. It also occurs over the tail and the neck, near the mane. It is disposed to spread, but not rapidly. The dry, light-colored scales are usually deepest in the center of the patches. The patches vary much in size. There is some itching, and sometimes, in chronic cases, cracks and suppuration also. The disease is aggravated by dirt, moisture, sudden atmospheric changes, and inappropriate food.

Remedy.—Mild purgatives. Soak scales in a solution of soda or potassium carbonate, followed by a coat of iodine. Oil of mercury, weak ointments of biniodide of mercury or chrysophanic acid are useful. Wood tar oils and oil of cade alternated with the foregoing in chronic cases. Alkalies, sulphites, phosphorus, arsenic internally. A triple compound of arsenic, iodine, and mercury is given by Professor Williams. Green and oleaginous food, with a liberal supply of linseed in it. Occasional diuretic.

For doses, see pages 13 to 29.

ELEPHANTIASIS (CHRONIC WEED, DERMAL AND SUBDERMAL HYPERTROPHY),

A thick, dark, wrinkled, tuberculate, insensible condition of the skin, is caused by excess of skin development. It usually involves the larger part of an entire limb, and is frequently the result of repeated attacks of inflammation of the lymphatic vessels of that limb, growing worse with each attack. It may follow one attack of lymphangitis (inflammation of the lymphatic glands). It is dry, leather-like, sometimes scaly, falls into folds, and in chronic cases may crack and suppurate. It causes much alteration of the limb, deformity, and impairment of motion. As the

SKIN DISEASES.

skin increases in thickness, the adjacent muscular parts show waste.

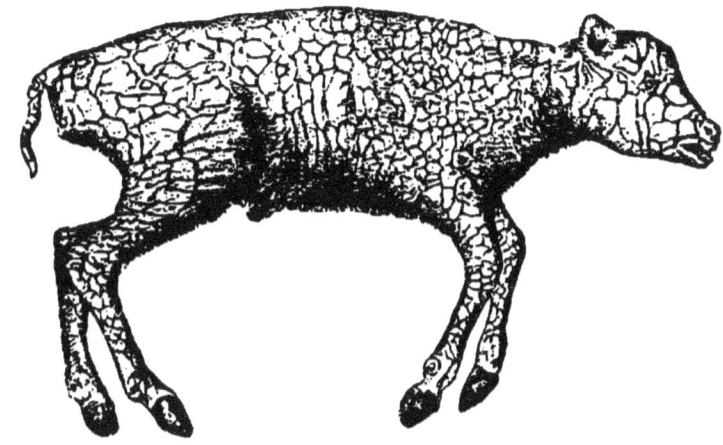

Fig. 42. Elephantiasis.

Remedy.—Usually only palliative. Laxatives, diuretics, salines, tonics—vegetable and mineral. Iodine, potassium iodide internally assist absorption. Mercurial or iodine ointment. Iron, copper salts, arsenic for debilitated. For doses, see pages 13 to 29.

PRURITUS (Itching, Nerve Disturbance, Perverted Sensibility),

Is local or general, the latter form being caused probably by some general disturbance. It is sometimes caused by parasites or other mites, but its cause is often insidious. It often appears suddenly and without warning. Except in very mild cases, pimples, pustules, corrugations, &c., appear, which, if rubbed or bitten, cause disfigurement, followed, after cure, by permanent blemishes. The disease seems to be affected by heat, moisture, and food.

Pruritus is regarded by some authorities as identical with Prurigo, but by Professor Robertson as a cutaneous neurosis (nerve disturbance), occurring independently of eruption or inflammation, and attacking both horses and dogs.

Remedy.—Where blood contamination is suspected, correct with general or special restoratives. For parasites rub in sulphur or sulphur iodide ointments, mercury oleate, carbolic or tar oils, stavesacre, or corrosive sublimate solutions. When resulting from sun heat, put in shade and wash with potassium bicarbonate; after which moisten spots with 2 parts glycerine, 1 each of sugar of lead and laudanum, 60 of water. Abate sensibility with hydrocyanic acid, potassium cyanide, or chloroform, alternated with alkaline washes. Purges, salines, careful diet when associated with gastric derangement. Iron salts, oleaginous food, alkalies, arsenic for debility.

GREASE (ERYSIPELATOUS IMPETIGO),

Is a disease of the cutaneous glands. The parts usually affected are the heels, especially the hind heels, where an unusual quantity of oily or lubricating substance is secreted. It is peculiar to lymphatic and coarsely bred and haired horses. It is caused by increased or perverted secretion, cold, moisture, perspiration, filth, indigestion, high feeding &c.

Symptoms.—Swelling; oily dripping; hair matted; soapy feel; bad odor; foot sensitive and stiff, but not much lameness. Swelling, sensitiveness, and lameness increase; exercise relieves latter.

Ulcerative stage: Disease extends half way up the leg, swelling increasing; pussy crusts form.

Grapy stage (described sometimes as a distinct disease): Grape-like clusters (also compared to coat of pine-apple) form, growing vascular, red, and sensitive; in chronic stage become cartilaginous and even horny; skin hard and thrice its natural thickness; most of the hair falls off; fetid, bloody, discharges from between grapes; increased swelling and lameness.

SKIN DISEASES.

Remedy.—Wash with soft or carbolic soap and warm water. Diuretics, salines, green food. Trim hair. Apply antiseptic bran poultice where there is much inflammation and discharge. Soak scabs with salicylic acid in solution

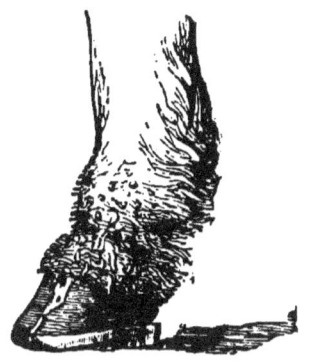

Fig. 43. First stage of confirmed Grease; exudative.

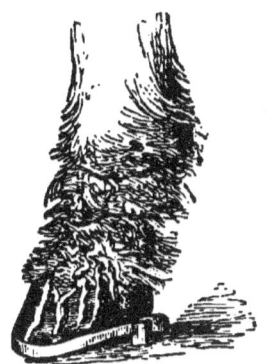

Fig. 44. Second stage; cracks.

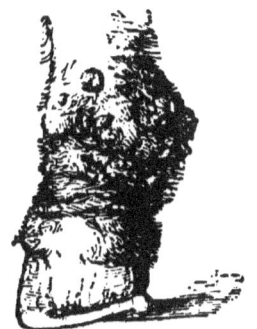

Fig. 45. Third stage; grapes.

of borax. Zinc sulphate, acetate, sulpho-carbolate, or chloride lotions, 3 parts to 100 of water, with 2 parts each of carbolic acid and glycerine. Vary dressing with sulphur iodide, wood tar oils, carbolic acid, or copper sulphate. Sulphuric acid and iron salts, iodine, arsenic internally. Remove the grapes with hot iron or caustics. Dress with solution of zinc sulphate or chloride or carbolic acid. For doses, see pages 13 to 29,

BALDNESS (ALOPECIA),

Is usually caused by disturbed nutrition and wasting changes of the skin and hair-cells. Parasites may or may not be present. It usually occurs suddenly, and is often extensive, with little or no irritation, itching, exudation, or swelling. The mane and tail are exempt. The bare skin is smooth, soft, and unctious, with a very slight covering of scales. The disease has a tendency to heal itself.

Remedy.—Oleaginous diet. General tonics, such as arsenic, iron, with gentian or nux vomica. Stimulate skin with ammonia liniment; cantharides tincture 1 part, soap or camphor liniment 8 parts; or castor oil. Shave, and rub in vaselin daily, dressing occasionally with the above stimulants. For doses, see pages 13 to 29.

LOUSINESS (PEDICULI, PHTHIRIASIS),

Is aided by damp dirt, barley straw, poverty, and privation. The horse suffers from three kinds of lice—two peculiar to itself, one peculiar to domestic fowl. The lice sometimes create such havoc that the hair falls off in places.

Remedy.—Wash with soft soap and warm water and rub in solution of stavesacre or tobacco, 1 part solution to 40 of water. Oil of tar 1 part, oil of rape or other mild oil 4 parts. Sulphur iodide ointment. Mercuric nitrate ointment. Use cautiously. Creosote 1 part, glycerine or alcohol 2 parts, water 40 parts. Clip long, coarse hair; isolate infected horses and cleanse premises.

MANGE, SCAB (SCABIES),

Is caused by several species of 'acari' (mange mites) burrowing under the skin. It is peculiar to unhealthy, unclean, coarse-bred, hairy-limbed horses and to cold weather. It is very contagious and requires isolation and careful treatment. A mangy horse will rub itself sore.

Symptoms.—The discovery of the insect, and the precise kind, is the best—is proof itself. Itching, rubbing, biting skin; hair falls off in patches; skin dry, white, lifeless, shedding scales and white dust and disclosing red pimples, and, in inveterate cases, becoming hard, dry, corrugated.

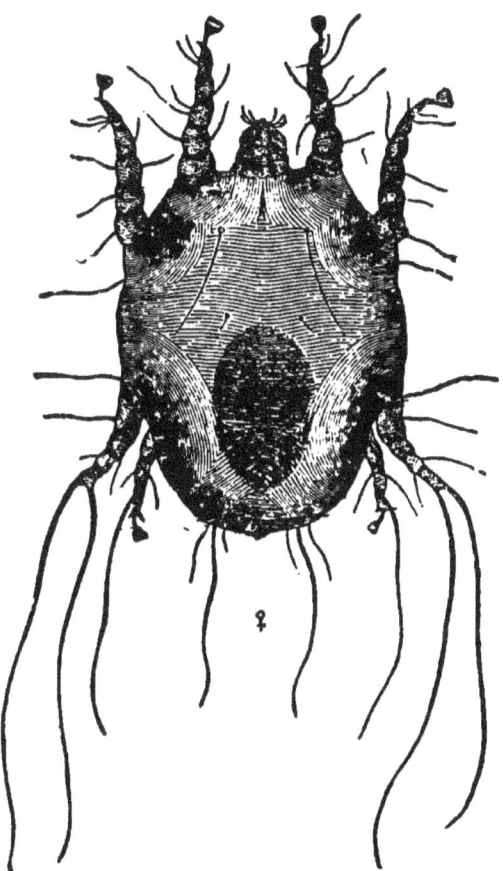

Fig. 46. The mite or acarus known as Symbiotes Equi. Magnified.

Remedy.—Wash: Cut up an ounce of common roll tobacco; keep in water near boiling point 6 to 12 hours; strain and make up 26 ounces, adding 2 to 4 ounces glycerine. Liniment: Linseed oil 1 pint, oil of tar 2 fluid ounces, sulphur 2 ounces. Rub one or other of these

170 THE DISEASES OF THE HORSE.

dressings in well for 2 days, to remain 3 or 4 days; then wash with soft soap and tepid water and reapply if nec-

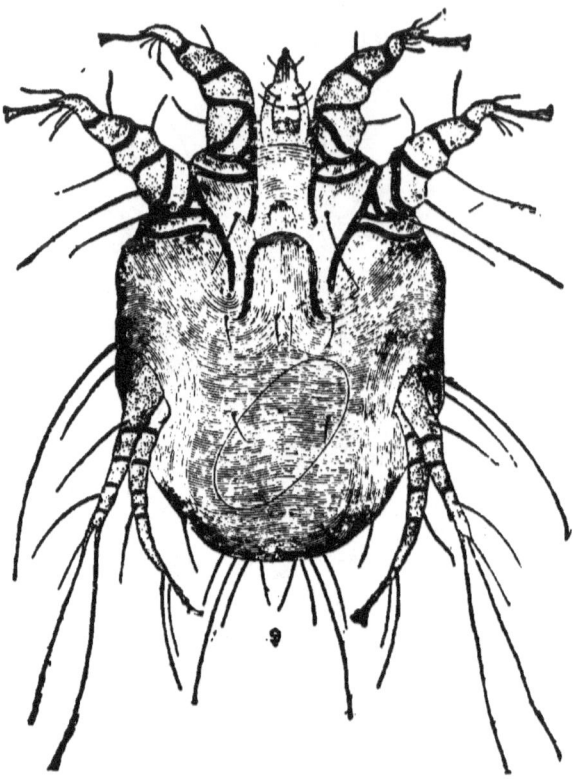

Fig. 47. The mite or acarus known as Dermatodectes Equi. Magnified.

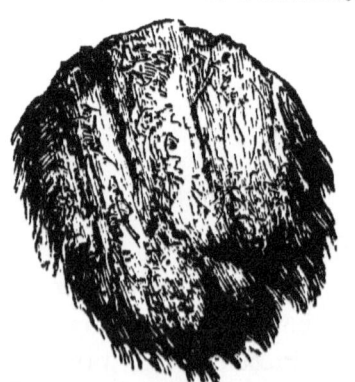

Fig. 48 A piece of mangy skin.

essary. Wash and disinfect with carbolic or corrosive sublimate solution clothing, harness, stable fittings, rubbing posts, &c.

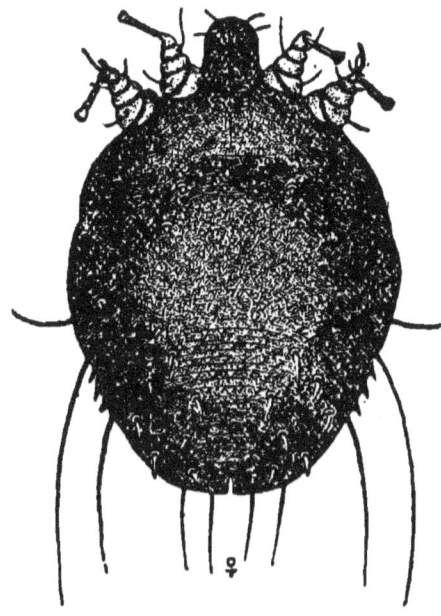

Fig. 49. The mite or acarus known as Sarcoptes Equi. Magnified.

RINGWORM OR TETTER (Proper),

Is caused by vegetable parasites (gnawing worms), which implant themselves in the hair follicles (secreting cells). Dampness, darkness, and improper diet favor their production. Young horses suffer most. The more or less circular patches are clear gray and shining. The hair falls out, disclosing either minute eruptions or distinct and separable scales. Some patches have healthy spots in the center, but it sometimes seems to cure itself through the death of the parasites.

Ringworm, Yellow or Honeycomb, is also caused by parasites, which may be transplanted to other animals. The patches consist of cup-shaped, yellowish scabs or crusts, sometimes separate, at others confluent. The odor

172   THE DISEASES OF THE HORSE.

is peculiar. It has been likened to that of bruised hemlock and mouse and cat's urine.

Remedy.—Soak and wash with lead subacetate solution 1 part to 90 of water. Then moderately paint with compound solution or tincture of iodine; or a smart application of common iodine ointment; or a thorough satura-

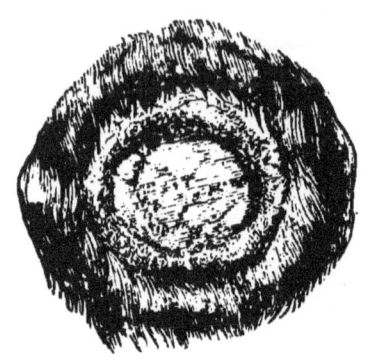

Fig. 50.   Ringworm.   Fig. 51.   Another specimen of same.

tion with corrosive sublimate, 2 to 4 grains to ounce of water, adding a little glycerine. Paraffin is good. Salines, tonics, arsenic internally, help to abate irritation and swelling. Soaking with oil softens and removes scales. Isolate. Disinfect brushes, harness, &c. No currying.

For doses, see pages 13 to 29.

SADDLE SCALD

Is sometimes hard to cure. The skin may be in an irritable condition, and therefore less able to stand the friction of the saddle and the acridity of the perspiration. From a slight, patchy excoriation, or perhaps only depilation, the skin of the back and sides will sooner or later become ulcerated, rendering the animal useless for saddle purposes.

Remedy.—Improve the fit of the saddle; line flaps with linen instead of serge, and make them more flexible and smaller if necessary. The medical means are purging and various local applications, such as are recommended for mangy affections (page 169).

HIDEBOUND

Is caused by lack of nutrition (health-giving food) indigestion, worms in the intestinal canal, chronic inflammation of the lungs, lack of exercise, exposure to cold, &c. Sometimes the ribs can be counted with the eye. Coat staring. The skin may be perfectly healthy.

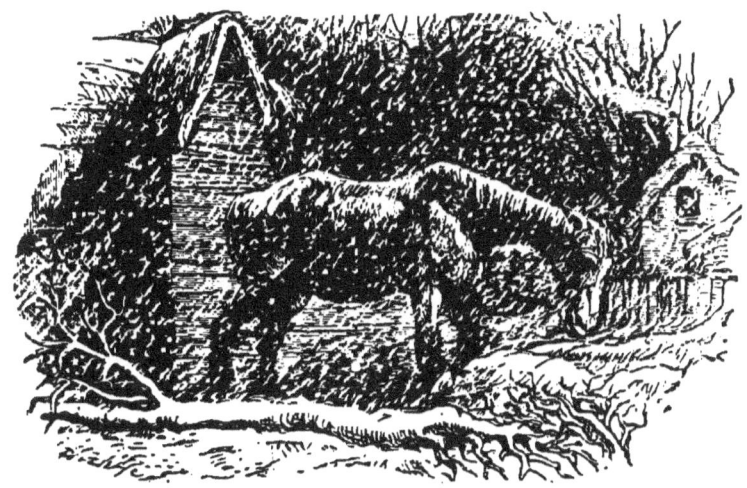

Fig. 52. One cause of Hidebound.

The remedy is nutritious food. If there is disease, cure it.

CRACKED HEEL

Is analogous in nature, cause, and remedy to grease, namely: It is peculiar to the hind legs, to coarse, fleshy. white legs, and cold, wet weather; consists in (transverse) ulcerations; the legs fill; the secretion is disordered, but the skin is stretched and cracked; remoteness of heel from the heart; motion of heel; secreting nature of surface; filth irritation; need of astringent applications, poultices, &c. Stopping thrush in feet will sometimes cause the heels to crack and break out in pimples. This is best counteracted by aperients and diuretics.

Remedy.—Treated according to origin, duration, and condition. When from wet ground, remove to dry; when from filth, *cool* and *fine* legs by cautious purging. If the ulceration has not penetrated through the skin, bran poultices, mild astringent powder, weak solutions of blue vitriol, alum, tincture of myrrh, benzoin, &c.; poultice best. If through skin, heroic treatment; slough with butter of antimony or nitric acid; some use lunar caustic or a red hot iron. Wipe dry; sprinkle caustic; poultice. High-heeled shoes if necessary. Watch frog. Overexercise injurious. Green food. (Percivall.)

SORENESS ABOUT THE ANUS.

There is a sort of eruption consisting of patchy excoriation and slight ulceration around the verge of the anus. It occurs usually in the spring, and is accompanied by costiveness. It is ascribed to a disordered alimentary canal, preternaturally hot, acrimonious fecal discharges, which increase the external irritation.

Remedy.—Wash twice a day, wipe dry, and sprinkle with common flour. Gentle purge if necessary.

WARTS (VERRUCÆ).

A horse may be so covered with warts as to be temporarily useless. Their most common situations are the head (eyelids, muzzle, ears), belly, sheath, penis, and inner side of thigh and arm. They are said to be produced by the skin, whence they derive their coverings. Some grow by pedicles; others have broad roots; others still are incased in the skin, out of which they slip, if pressed, when freed by the knife. Some are no larger than peas, others as large as marbles or walnuts, while a single wart has been known to grow till it impeded the action of a limb. They are usually enveloped in thin, smooth, and hairless skin, but which in time becomes callous and horny. Others are ulcerous and even fungoid, bleeding on the least irritation and showing no disposition to heal. Internally they exhibit a firm, fibro-cartilaginous texture, little or no vascularity, and seldom bleed except from their roots.

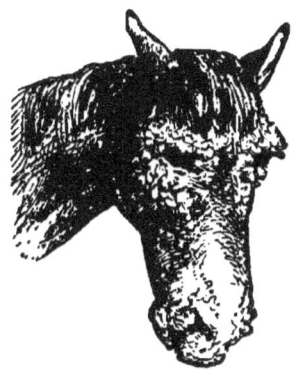

Fig. 53. Warts.

Remedy.—Remove by excision, torsion, or ligature. To prevent return, cauterize the site of those about the penis. Chromic acid, silver nitrate, and glacial acetic acid destroy warts. The soft variety gradually removed by daily moistening with commercial acetic acid.

Where the wart grows from a slender pedicle, a double, well waxed, silk ligature, drawn tightly, is the best means of removal. Should the ligature cut the wart, apply the budding iron to its surface. Encysted warts require crucial incisions and pressing only. If a wart has a broad base, caustic is more effectual than ligature. Sprinkle the wart with arsenic. It will fall off in about two weeks. Sulphur made into a paste, with sulphuric acid, will answer the same purpose. Chloride of zinc, powdered, and rubbed with a simple ointment, is good. Warts of the eyelids should be removed with the knife.

Greasiness of the Skin.—Percivall describes the case of a horse, recently returned from grass, which, while shedding its coat in September, showed an exceedingly greasy condition of the skin. It was washed with soft soap, but in three days became greasy again. A week afterward, after giving a fourth dose of physic, the animal was washed in water in which an alkali had been dissolved.

INJURIES.

Injuries are mechanical, chemical, and mixed. Mechanical injuries comprehend wounds, contusions, abrasions, fractures, dislocations, &c. Chemical injuries are caused by heat, the concentrated acids, caustic alkalies, lunar caustic, corrosive sublimate, arsenic, &c. Mixed injuries are caused by the bites or stings of mad dogs, insects, &c. Also from inoculation.

WOUNDS

Are incised, contused, lacerated, punctured, gun-shot, and poisoned. The first danger, especially in incised wounds, is bleeding, the remedy for which is (1) a ligature; (2) a tourniquet or, what is better, a rubber band; (3) trickling water; (4) pressure (a compress if practica-

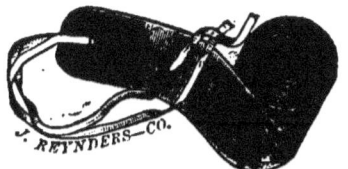

Fig. 54. Rubber Bandage.

ble); (5) styptics, such as tow, lint, matico, ergot, digitalis, ice, lead acetate.

Blood from a vein is dark colored, and flows in an uninterrupted and comparatively tardy stream. Ligatures should be withdrawn in 10 or 14 days, or they will fester. Cut the thread.

The bleeding stopped, the next thing after the removal

of foreign bodies and clots of blood, is washing with one of the following antiseptics: 1. Carbolic acid 1 part with 20 to 40 of water. 2. Corrosive sublimate 1 part, common salt 7½, water, 1,000. 3. Zinc chloride 1 part, water 80 to 100. 4. Mercuric iodide and potassium iodide each 1 part, water 1,000. 5. Hydronaphtol 1 part, rectified spirit 1 part, water 300. 6. Sodium hydrofluosilicate 1 part, water 500. The latter is "a recently discovered, effectual, non-poisonous, cheap germicide." (Dun.)

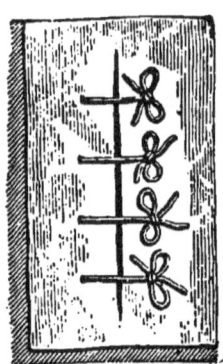

Fig. 55. Interrupted Suture.

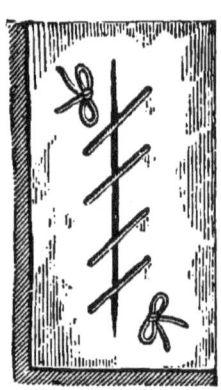

Fig. 56. Uninterrupted Suture.

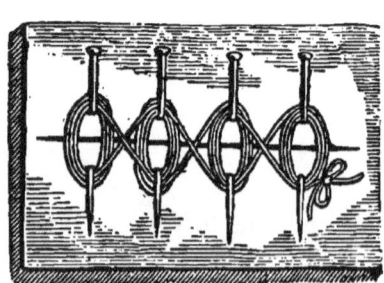

Fig. 57. Twisted Suture.

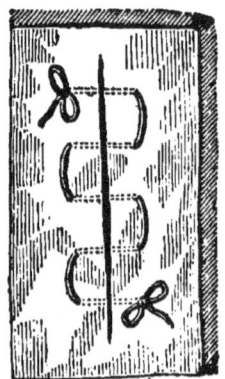

Fig. 58. Zigzag Suture.

Incised wounds are brought together by sutures (stitches) pins, or plasters. Bandages keep the parts in apposition and give support. Splints and slings are sometimes required.

In large contused or lacerated wounds a dependent opening must be made by drainage tubes or otherwise. Deeply punctured and lacerated wounds are fomented for some hours in order to limit inflammation. Apply a sheet of carbolic lint, on which either place a poultice or let cold water trickle over it.

Superficial wounds heal by first intention (without pus) when the edges are held together by plaster, styptic colloid, or shellac, applied in methylated spirit (90 parts of rectified spirit (alcohol), 10 parts of wood spirit, or impure methylic alcohol.)

Poisoned wounds are treated according to their nature. Poison may be kept out of the circulation by ligature. Excision of the poisoned textures may be desirable, and also subsequent cauterization or irrigation with a suitable germicide.

Wounds properly closed and healing satisfactorily should not be disturbed except for cleansing and redressing. Do not be in a hurry about removing sutures.

If a wound becomes inflamed or painful, or the discharges are unhealthy, remove the dressings, cut the sutures, remove blood clots or other irritants, irrigate or

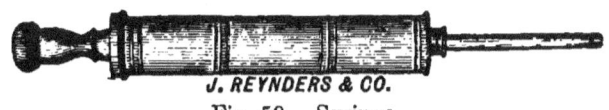

Fig. 59. Syringe.

syringe the surfaces with an antiseptic, and apply a poultice over the carbolic lint if necessary. Use opium and belladonna with poultices or antiseptics when there is much pain.

Excessive granulation checked by pressure, astringents, or occasional use of caustics.

A dose of physic, cooling, digestible diet, and healthful

surroundings are essential to the successful treatment of wounds.

INJURED EYES.

Blows are usually received on the orbital process (bony projection), when the ball of the eye is rarely injured. In such cases the upper eyelid is usually swollen and the outer membrane of the eye itself may partake of it. Wet and apply a linen cloth, or sponge the part as often as it becomes dry. In cases of extreme swelling, local bleeding and fomentations will be effective.

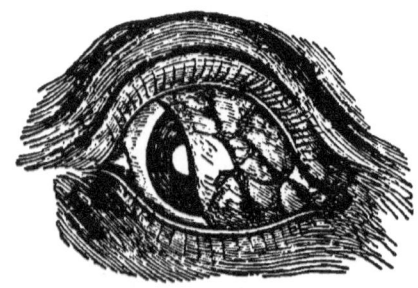

Fig. 60. The haw (the horse's handkerchief).

When hayseeds, insects, dirt, &c., get under the upper lids, and the haw fails to expel them, turn back the lid and remove them by hand.

Cuts and lacerations sometimes penetrate the ball. If they extend through the cornea, the watery fluid will escape and the iris protrude. Return the iris carefully. Foment with warm water in which poppy heads have been boiled. After this, apply healing washes with a camel's hair pencil. Shade the eye.

Laceration of the Eyelid is not an uncommon accident. It may be caused by a bite, a nail, hook, &c. It usually begins at the inner, superior, and most projecting part of the lid, but the reverse may be the case. The wound usually causes considerable bleeding.

Remedy.—Secure the horse, cleanse the eye, and stitch

with strong sewing silk, using a small, sharp, crooked needle. In a week or so, or as soon as the parts cohere, or when pus oozes out, cut and withdraw the stitches. After this it is important to secure the horse with double straps, otherwise, owing to the irritation of the eye, it will rub against the stall and dissever the parts.

INJURIES TO MOUTH, TONGUE, JAWS.

The tongue may be injured in various ways. It may be bitten accidentally by the horse itself, also, when protruded, by another horse; by sharp projections of the teeth, rough or careless usage, &c. Stitch the parts together whenever necessary and practicable, cleanse the wound if necessary, and leave the healing to nature.

The branches of the lower jaw are common seats of fracture, a frequent cause of which is the use of sharp-curved bits, but rough usage will sometimes cause fractures even with a smooth bit. The horse loses its appetite and is unfit for work. The fractured bone must be removed, but it is often better to wait a week or ten days that nature may loosen the parts. Fractures are often the result of external violence. A severe blow in the region of the roots of the teeth may cause a fracture that will necessitate the removal of both bone and teeth.

The jaw is also subject to injury from violence with the curb-rein. The outside gum is squeezed by the crub. An abscess forms within the bone, and there is usually sooner or later bone to be removed. Keep the wound open and encourage the discharge. A scruple of hydrochloric acid in an ounce of water is a good dressing. If the horse must be worked, use a snaffle.

The outside of the lips and cheeks are sometimes severely cut by sharp and twisted snaffles, the inside of the cheek by sharp projections of the molar teeth. The only remedy for the latter is to file the projections down, but not so as to destroy the natural slant of the grinding surface, as already explained on page 142. The checks will heal without aid, but an ounce of alum in a quart of water is a good wash for them.

SADDLE-GALLS, SITFASTS, WARBLES, TUMOR ON THE ELBOW.

These injuries are caused by pinching of the harness-pad, girths, or collar, bad-fitting or overweighted saddles, &c. If they are neglected or exposed to further injury, they either turn to abscesses or subside into smaller tumors and are indisposed to undergo further change, though they are sometimes carried off by suppuration. Percivall says that when a bad-fitting saddle has been kept on too long and evil results are expected, that it should be allowed to remain on the back till the horse is perfectly cool.

Cure saddle-gall by removal of cause. Bathe and cleanse once a day; hot water if suppurating. Antiseptic dressings. Swollen fatty follicles reduced with soap liniment; in chronic cases foment and lance.

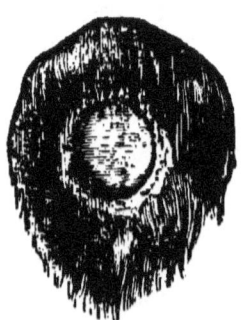

Fig. 61. Sitfast.

Sitfast is "a part of a horse's back turned horny." To use another simile, repeated injury by the saddle causes the formation of horny excrescences resembling corns of the human foot. The sitfast acquires a well defined border. In many instances the skin withdraws from around it, and a little matter oozes from between it and the skin. This indicates that the sitfast will be carried off by sloughing. If the process is slow, it may be hastened by blistering ointment. Dissect out if necessary.

Warbles or grubs "are small, hard tumors on the saddle part of a horse's back;" also the neck and sometimes the tail. When recent they yield to stimulating lotions, though sometimes they run on to suppuration and disperse. Frequently, however, they become callous, in which condition they may continue for years without serious consequences. They may be dissected out.

According to Williams warbles in the ox is caused by a bot-fly which lodges under the skin.

Tumor on the elbow (shoeboil) is caused by contusion or pressure of the heel of the fore shoe or by the horse lying on a hard pavement with insufficient bedding.

INFLAMED VEIN (PHLEBITIS),

Is usually the result of bleeding, but some horses are predisposed to it. It is also the result of violence after bleeding—disturbing the pin by rubbing against this or that. Injury may also follow from using an unclean or rusty instrument in bleeding. The wound should be speedily closed. The lips, unless disturbed, will rarely fail to adhere. Tie the horse's head up to prevent rubbing. If worked, guard against injury by either bridle rein or collar.

Remedy.—Open any abscesses. If swelling occurs while the pin is in, withdraw it carefully so as not to disturb the wound. Foment and poultice. Laxative diet. If the wound is foul and the vein corded up to the head, leave the orifice open and apply a blister, renewing it as often as needed. If necessary, the vein may be tied. In case of fresh bleeding, pin or stitch and compress the wound, keeping the head tied up. A horse with an impervious jugular should not be turned to grass. Diffuse phlebitis treated antiseptically, with salines internally. For a list of antiseptics and salines, see pages 31 and 36 respectively.

LACERATED KNEE

Is usually a much more serious injury than a contused or bruised knee, for it may penetrate to and even expose the knee joint. The extent or depth of the wound is a matter of great importance, for the treatment must be regulated by it. The healing of the wound requires time and patience, for the part is much used and the skin thereby stretched.

The accident is usually the result of tenderness and lameness of the fore legs, tripping, cutting, and unequal action, rough roads and pavements, rolling stones, &c.

The scar left is sometimes quite a blemish. Ordinary scars may be removed by blistering the part, first shaving off the hair.

Remedy.—Cleanse the part thoroughly with warm water and allay inflammation by fomentation. Use a cradle for a few days to prevent the part from being bitten. If the knee does not heal kindly, apply lotions or poultices. After this dress with tincture of benzoin or compound tincture of myrrh. Toward the end, a solution of blue vitriol may be needed. In place of the two last, after poulticing, sprinkle daily with a powder of flour and alum. In some cases it may be advisable to stitch the skin together. Quiet. Sling if necessary.

OPEN KNEE AND OTHER JOINTS.

A joint must be penetrated to constitute this injury, but even if it is not penetrated, it is often opened by sloughing. It is a very serious matter, for the joint oil (synovia) often escapes, causing a stiff joint (anchylosis). The discharge of oil, however, does not necessarily indicate opened joint, for the sheaths of the tendons contain an oil precisely like joint oil. Tetanus (commonly called lock-jaw) may result from the injury. Opened joint is usually caused by a fall, but it may be caused by a thorn, a nail, or a sharp-pointed instrument.

Symptoms.—Knee clotted with dirt and blood; foot rests on toe, not because the joint is painful, for recently injured joints have little or no sensation, but because of the painful ligaments, tendons, &c. In a day the parts are hot, full, and tender, these symptoms increasing from day to day. About this time the constitution sympathizes; fever; pulse rises; appetite and spirits lost; mouth dry; eyes injected; skin and limbs warm; breathing disturbed. The animal now exchanges its dull mood for watching and irritability. If the irritation is not checked, it is likely to exhaust the vital energies before the local inflammation even turns toward restoration.

Remedy.—Cleanse and foment. Antiseptic dressing. Stitch, if the movement of the joint and tearing loose can be prevented. Styptic colloid, collodion, or plaster for support and protection. Splints and bandages. Sling or tie up to prevent lying down. Half doses of physic; cooling diet. Let a weak antiseptic solution trickle over a calico bandage lightly laid over the joint. Blister if necessary.

WOUNDED TENDONS

Are usually caused by thorns, stubs, flints, kicks, treads, &c. If properly treated, they usually end well. A tendon may be even severed, and yet be restored by approximation. Thorns have been known to work themselves out between skin and hoof. Some fester and discharge themselves. Some are sloughed out with medicines. In some cases the parts around the foreign substance become hardened and continue so without lameness. It is possible for tetanus to follow wounded tendons.

Remedy.—Fomentations, poultices, cooling lotions. Loosen as well as cool part. Sling. Splints, starch bandages. When inflammation has moderated, stimulate externally.

INFLAMED LYMPHATICS

The office of the lymphatic system is to form and circulate lymph. When disturbed, it is usually the result of wounds or pricks.

Remedy.—Remove cause. Cooling diet. Salines; potassium iodide. Foment while heat and tenderness continue; after which apply friction, bandages, iodine ointment. Continue salines in drinking water.

For doses, see pages 13 to 29.

STRAIN OF LOINS (PSOÆ) MUSCLES

Is caused by any injury that violently extends them. It is liable to be confounded with 'broken back,' from which it is distinguished by the animal being able to bend and extend the limbs. In some cases the animal almost drags its limbs.

Remedy.—Rugs wrung out of hot water applied over loins and abdomen. Anodyne injections (opium, morphine, &c.) Slings if both sides are affected.

BRUSHING OR INTERFERING

Occurs in horses with faulty action, especially when tired or out of condition. The part struck is the fetlock.

Remedy.—A ¾ shoe, or a shoe thin on inside web, without heel on outside. Boot on injured fetlock. Careful shoeing. Improve general condition.

SPEEDY-CUT

Is a bruise in the inner part of the limb, near the knee, caused by the opposite foot. Cause—round, high action (stepping). The horse is liable to fall from the violence of the blow.

Remedy.—Fomentations; open any abscess; antiseptic dressing. Prevent by reducing inner crust of offending foot, using nicely fitting ¾ shoes, removing shoes every 3 weeks. Protect leg with boot. Travel slowly.

SPRAIN OF MUSCLES, TENDONS, AND LIGAMENTS.

The fibers are severely stretched and in serious cases some of them are torn.

Remedy.—Rest; foment; purge. Slings in bad cases. When the tenderness and pain are abated, apply counter-

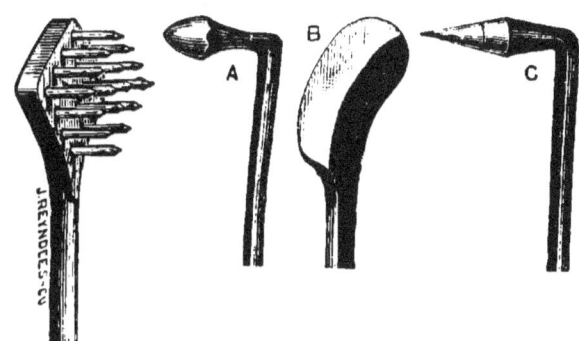

Fig. 62. Firing-Irons.

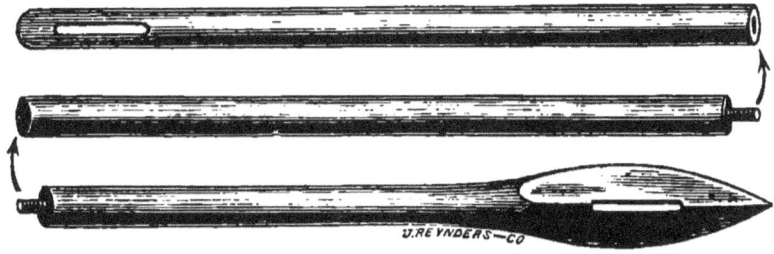

Fig. 63. Three-jointed, sharp Seton Needle.

irritants. Cantharides or mercuric iodide ointments. Firing-iron. Seton.

RUPTURED TENDONS OR LIGAMENTS.

Remedy.—Fomentations allay inflammation. Treat as for fractured bones. Quiet. Splints. Starch bandages. Slings. When inflammation moderates, stimulate externally.

PRICKED FOOT

Is caused by misdirected or defective nails in shoeing, nails picked up in walking, sharp instruments, flints, glass, &c. The injury will vary with the cause, the part injured, and the depth and direction of the wound. In shoeing if a nail causes blood to flow, lameness will soon follow; but if it only goes close to the quick, it may be one or even two weeks before lameness results.

Remedy.—Remove shoe and diseased tissue. Give pus vent by dependent opening. Inject with spirit turpentine. Keep hole free of dirt. Poultice.

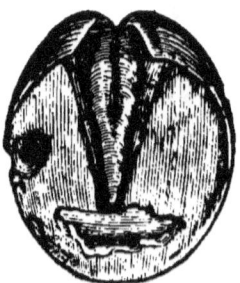

Fig. 64. Side puncture represents Pricked Foot, the front Bruised Sole.

BRUISE OF THE SOLE

Leads to the effusion of blood, but seldom causes serious lameness. Pare off the discolored horn and shoe at least once with leather. Treat as for 'Corns,' which see.

BRUISES (General).

Treat general bruises as follows: Foment, poultice, water dressing, refrigerants; carbolic acid and other antiseptics. Hand rubbing and subsequent rubbing with oil promote absorption. Lead, zinc and other astringent solutions probably prevent leucocytes (white cells) exuding. Belladonna, opium, aconite paralyze sensory nerves and relieve pain.

TREAD AND OVERREACH

Are identical in nature. A tread is a contused wound of the coronet of either the hind or fore foot, caused by the opposite foot. An overreach is a tread on the coronet of the fore foot by the hind foot. The parts injured consist of skin, cartilage, and horn. The injury is therefore complex and requires careful treatment.

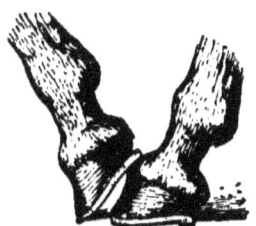 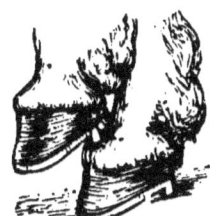 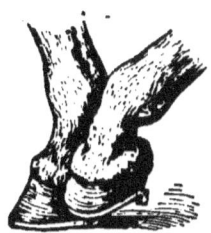

Fig. 65. Tread.   Fig. 66. Tread.   Fig. 67. Overreach.

Remedy.—Remove hair and such lacerated parts of horn as may harbor dirt. Immerse in warm water. Hot poultice, but discontinue when healing begins. Turpentine or nitric acid lotion dressing. Physic. Heels of shoes well rounded off. Light shoes. Protect coronet with pad.

FROST BITE (GELATIO),

If often repeated, causes the part to become permanently weakened, slightly swelled, of a purple color, with less heat, and afterward inflamed. The skin cracks, and a discharge of sanguineous matter takes place. More intense cold entirely suspends vital action, the part becoming pale, insensible, and shriveled. The skin, especially the heel, will often slough across from side to side, forming a strip of dead skin, under which is a deep chasm, called a cracked heel.

Remedy.—Raise temperature of frozen parts gradually.

Stimulants to affected parts; turpentine and oil; soap liniment. Treat sloughs antiseptically.

QUITTOR

Is a sore or wound on the coronet connected with a sinus (cavity) in the foot, the sinus running between the sensitive parts and the horn. It is usually caused by the large, awkward calkins of the hind shoe, but any neglected wound of the coronet may cause it. It may also be caused by an abscess within the foot; also by a festered corn.

The disease at first is insidious, being covered by the hair. When the tumor points, the hair falls off and reveals the cause of the lameness.

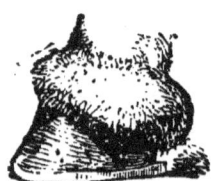 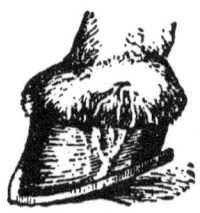

Fig. 68. Quittor before pus exudes through coronet.   Fig. 69. Quittor after exudation through coronet.

In severe cases of quittor the skin, tendons, cartilages, and bones are more or less affected. When the bone becomes carious there is little hope of cure. A cure, even in ordinary cases, requires two or three months. The horse is usually lame even after the healing. This is owing to change of structure. The cartilage becoming bony and the coronet destroyed, often causes the disorder known as 'False Quarter.' Caries of either the cartilage or bone is preceded by ulcers having a greenish discharge mixed with synovia (joint oil).

Remedy.—Secure a free dependent opening. Remove dead tissues or other irritants. Poultice. Inject corrosive sublimate solution. Where cavities are numerous and difficult of access, core them out with corrosive sublimate or arsenic plug. Where foot is strong, no shoe is needed; if weak or broken, bar shoe relieves pressure. In very bad cases diseased textures must be excised. Blister coronet to promote reparative action.

FALSE QUARTER

Results from quittor more than from any other cause. It may, however, be caused by injury or disease of any kind destroying the coronary substance, on the integrity of which the integrity of the wall depends. In the same way that injury at the root of man's nails causes division, will injury of the coronary substance cause a groove in the hoof. Hence the name. Its appearance is that of a gap. The gap is covered with a thin layer of soft horn,

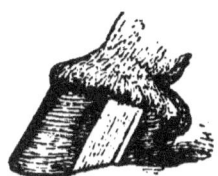

Fig. 70. False Quarter.

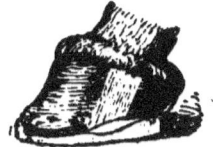

Fig. 71. Remedy for False Quarter.

which sometimes splits and bleeds. Dirt or squeezing of the internal parts sometimes causes inflammation, pus, and lameness. If the fissure remains sound, however, no inconvenience follows. False quarter may be palliated, but not cured.

Remedy.—Restore secretory function of coronary band. Dress and promote healing of any wounds in band. Pressure should generally be applied and dead horn trimmed away. Bar shoe to relieve concussion. Fill cracks with gutta-percha to keep out dirt. Blisters to coronet sometimes useful.

VENOMOUS BITES AND STINGS

Are caused by bees, hornets, vipers, &c. The adder's bite is sometimes fatal, and swarming bees have been known to sting a horse or ox to death.

Remedy.—Ammonia and oil; or an ounce of spirit of hartshorn or turpentine in olive oil. Rub some on bite also. Potassium hydrate or bicarbonate solutions. Bathe the eyes with laurel water twice a week. Carbolic acid; prussic acid; chloroform; cold water dressings. For snake bite ligature limb; excise wound, and sear with hot iron. Alcoholic stimulants; ammonia. Artificial respiration.

For doses, see pages 13 to 29.

BURNS AND SCALDS.

Remedy.—Protect immediately from air and irritants by layers of cotton wool, or apply carron oil. Liniment of oil and litharge, with 5 per cent. boric, salicylic, or carbolic acid, or peppermint oil. Whiting and water, or Fuller's earth, about the consistence of cream, applied till well coated. Zinc oxide, with about 10 parts vaselin, or of glycerine and water. Alkaline solutions, soap lather, saturated solution sodium bicarbonate for slighter cases. Where discharges are foul, add antiseptics to above dressings. Where there is irritation and pain, add chloroform or laudanum, or both. Combat constitutional suffering with antiseptics and anodynes internally. For doses, see pages 13 to 29. For lists of antiseptics, anodynes, &c., see pages 30 to 37.

FRACTURES

Are usually caused by blows, falls, slips, &c., but a horse, by struggling when cast, may not only fracture its spine but perhaps some other bone.

Fractures are simple, compound, or comminuted; they are also either transverse or oblique. They are indicated by a grating noise; separation or displacement of the parts; deformity, shortening, lameness; pain on pressure; heat, swelling, tension, or the approach of inflammation. The three chief principles of treatment are replacement, maintainment, and care.

Compound and comminuted fractures are hopeless. Reducible simple fractures are sometimes curable, such as fracture of the ribs, cannon bones, arch of orbit, nasal bones, upper and lower jaw bones, tail bones, arm, hock, leg, pastern, and coffin (foot) bones.

The following fractures are usually fatal: Skull, pelvis, spine, scapula, humerus, femur, tibia, elbow, patella (stifle bone), and the sesamoid (foot), coronary, and navicular bones.

Repeated displacements and indisposition to form callus (bony substance between fractured parts) are also incurable.

Remedy.—Put bones in apposition. Splints of leather, lath, block-tin, paroplastic, or gutta-percha. Incase in plaster of Paris; starch bandages. Ends of bones may be kept together by metallic sutures. Smart blister causes outpouring of fibrinous, plastic, reparative material; also favors parts being kept at rest. Large animals may require slinging. Wounds in compound fractures treated antiseptically. Calcium phosphate internally in weakly subjects hastens union. For doses, see pages 13 to 29.

DISLOCATIONS

Occur less frequently than fractures and are usually less remediable. They are either complete or partial. They are caused by blows, falls, wrenches, &c., or by violent action of muscles. In some cases these causes seem to cooperate. Replacement, retention, and care are necessary to recovery.

The spine, especially at the neck, and the scapula and hip are sometimes successfully replaced.

Stifle dislocation is common and is easily remedied. 1.

Back the horse forcibly and suddenly and somewhat diagonally a few paces. 2. If the first remedy does not succeed, fix a line around the pastern, the other end passed over the neck. Pull the limb forward till the fetlock is nearly as high as the elbow on the same side. Press the bone forward and inward with a jerk. If the displacement is inward, which is rare and cannot occur without great violence, if the hand is not strong enough, press the bone upward and outward with a piece of wood.

To prevent a recurrence of the dislocation, keep the horse quiet—in a sling if necessary—applying stimulants, blisters, or plasters. A wide bandage, with a hole in the middle for the patella (stifle), and laced behind the limb, may be successfully applied, especially if the skin is made adhesive with Canada balsam. Keep the limb extended with a line around the pastern and neck.

Abate inflammation in all dislocations by hot fomentations or cold water.

The symptoms of dislocation are: Change in the appearance of the dislocated part—depression at joint, prominence and tenderness at the then place of lodgment; peculiar noise and acute pain in moving the part; considerable swelling. Compare the dislocated part with the opposite side.

When the stifle is dislocated, the symptoms, in addition to the above, are: Backward protrusion of limb; pastern and foot bent to utmost; cannot be straightened; limb trailed, describing the segment of a circle when the animal moves.

LAMENESSES.

CANKER

Is a constitutional disease of the feet, and is due to a habit of body or grossness of constitution, as exhibited by thick, round legs, large feet, and the lymphatic temperament. It usually begins in the frog, but it may begin in any other part of the plantar surface. It much resembles grease of the leg, and often coexists with it. There is an abundant, fetid, colorless discharge from the frog, which is large, spongy, and covered by pallid, stringy

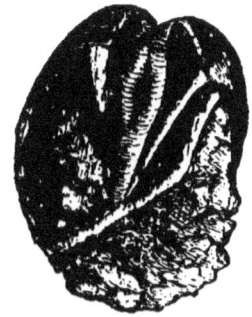
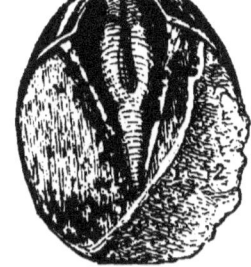

Fig. 72. Worst stage of Canker. Fig. 73. Improvement in Canker.

prominences of a fungoid nature, intermixed with an offensive smelling, semi-dried, cheesy matter, composed of imperfect horn cells. The sound feet of a horse predisposed to canker very often have an abominable smell, as if the animal suffered from a "sulphureted hydrogen diathesis." (Williams.)

Remedy.—Remove all superfluous horn and fungous growths. Dress with silver nitrate, chromic acid, zinc chloride solution, or sulphuric acid and tar. In persistent cases caustics and astringents must be changed frequently. Tonics and salines. Liberal diet. Cleanliness. Pressure to fetlock for bleeding. Pack with dry tow; bandage; protect with leather boot. For doses, see pages 13 to 29.

THRUSH

Is a fetid discharge from the frog. The cleft is usually first affected. If neglected the disease spreads over the whole organ, the horn becoming detatched from the bulbs of the heels to the toe of the frog. The cause is usually filth, but the disease may originate in frost-bite, grease, swelled legs, &c.

Thrush differs from canker in the nature of the diseased secretion, and also in its course and tractability.

Remedy.—Cleanliness. A leather sole may be placed within the shoe. Dust with calomel. Dress with tar or wood tar oil. Dose of physic, especially when associated with constitutional causes. Regulate feeding and work. Shoe with tips if feet strong and animal works chiefly on land.

BONE SPAVIN

Is a bony tumor on the inner and lower part of the hock, arising from inflammation of the cuneiform and metatarsal bones, terminating usually in stiffness of one or more of the gliding joints of the hock. It is very rare on the outer side of the hock.

Spavins arise from causes that are hereditary or constitutional and local. The local or exciting causes are sprains of the ligaments and concussion of the bones. One fertile cause is the alteration of the direction of the leg, induced by the use of high calkined shoes. These high heels alter the relative position of the limb, from the hip downward, and cause shocks of concussion at every step.

Remedy.—Rest. Purgative and fomentations where

there is much lameness. In young horses hasten the inevitable stiffness by a blister, firing, seton, or periosteotomy (dividing the periosteum, a very hard, elastic substance next to the bones and roots of the teeth). In old horses sometimes incurable. The bone softens.

BOG SPAVIN,

When caused by inflammation of the joint, is a tense, fluctuating swelling, accompanied by heat and pain. This form constitutes unsoundness. It may be acute or chronic. In the acute form the lameness is very great, with fever, loss of condition, and the ability to put the foot to the ground. It is apt to end in ulceration of the articular

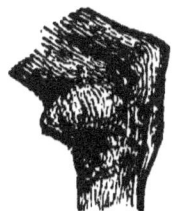

Fig. 74. Bog Spavin, or distention of the chief synovial membrane of the hock joint.

cartilage and partial stiffness of the joint. Some bog spavins, however, are almost harmless, being mere dropsy of the articulation (synovia for lubricating joints), arising from some fault of conformation.

Remedy.—Rest; in severe cases sling. High heeled shoe. Foment when hot and tender. Cold water and refrigerants when inflammation abates. Spring truss in young animals sometimes gives equable pressure. Counter-irritation encourages absorption. Firing-iron or seton in chronic cases.

THOROUGH-PIN OF THE HOCK

Is a small, roundish or oval, membranous cavity on the lower part of the thigh and upper and back part of the hock, caused by disease of the tendon of the flexor pedis perforans muscle, which muscle is inclosed in a synovial sheath on the inner side of the 'os calcis,' or by dropsy of the sheath itself, without disease of the tendon. The fluid which fills it may, by pressure, be forced from one side to the other. Hence the name thorough-pin (through and through). This may be described as true thorough-pin, in contradistinction to that associated with very large bog spavins. Thorough-pin is peculiar to short, fleshy, upright hocks.

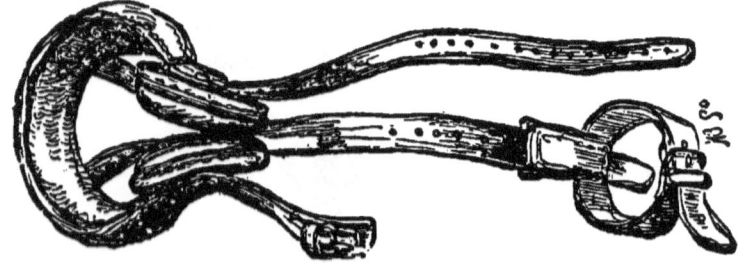

Fig. 75. Spring Truss for Thorough-pin and Bog Spavin.

Remedy.—Rest; high heeled shoe; flannel bandages. Equable pressure from a spring truss. Blister if swelling persists. Open sac at most dependent part if necessary.

THOROUGH-PIN OF THE KNEE

Consists in swelling of the sheath containing the perforatis and perforans tendons, at the back and a little above the knee joint, and is treated similarly to thorough-pin of the hock.

SPLINT

Is a bony tumor (exostosis), usually, when on the fore feet, on the inner surface of the metatarsal or metacarpal bones. Splint of the hind feet, however, is usually on the outer surface of the metatarsal bone. It seldom causes lameness in the hind feet, and does not always cause it in the fore.

Splint is caused by concussion and hereditary predisposition, especially that arising from shape and form of leg. The effects of concussion may be due to the immature age of the bone, shape of leg, method of shoeing, or overwork or speed when young.

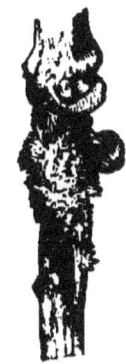

Fig. 76. Splints (fine points of bone).

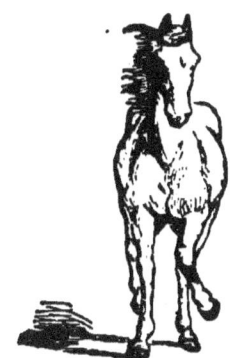

Fig. 77. "Dishing," while on the trot, caused by irritation from fine-points of bone.

Remedy.—In slight cases stop fast work. Half dose physic. Foment and then blister. In severe cases periosteotomy. Pyro-puncture preferable to firing, as it does not blemish. Mercuric iodide ointment usually reduces deposit.

STRINGHALT (CHOREA),

Is a spasmodic movement of the muscles of the limbs, usually the hind.

Incurable. Remove any spavin or other adverse condition. Temporary benefit results from a laxative, a course of bromides, and moderate work. Stretching and section of the tibial nerves are of no avail.

Other muscles are subject to spasmodic action, especially those of the spine.

CURB

Is a sprain or injury of the straight ligament of the hock, causing enlargement of the joint. It is apt to cause lameness in young horses, and, when of fresh origin, in horses of any age. But when of long standing, and merely the result of former disease, lameness rarely ensues. The form of hock the reverse of that liable to thorough-pin is the one predisposed to curb.

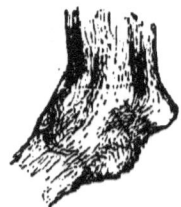 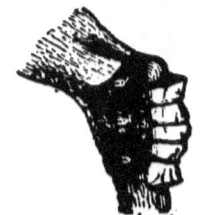

Fig. 78. Curb. Fig. 79. India-rubber bandage for keeping wet cloths on Curb.

Remedy.—Foment; lead acetate solution; refrigerants. Counter-irritants; mercuric or iodide ointment; charges (plasters). High heeled shoe; no toe pieces. Rest for several months, especially in young horses.

CORNS

Are bruises of the secreting sole. They occur almost invariably on the inside heel of the fore feet, and are

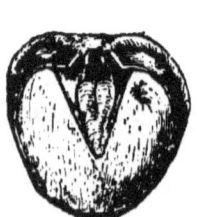 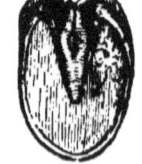 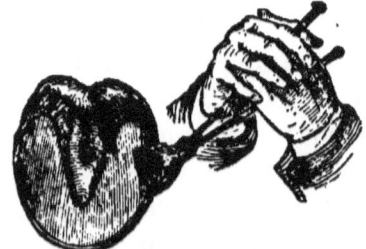

Fig. 80. Old Corn. Fig. 81. New Corn. Fig. 82. Test for Corns.

caused by bad shoeing. They are not horn tumors, but

may become such. Sometimes they end in suppuration, partial necrosis, or bony spiculæ.

Remedy.—Remove shoe, pare to relieve pressure and insure exit of pus. Poultices soften sole and abate tenderness. Use light shoe with wide web. Shoe strong feet with tips.

FOUNDER (LAMINITIS),

Is inflammation of the feet. It is a dreadful disease, and may be caused by concussion as well as gastric derangement (overeating). It is sometimes communicated to the feet by other diseases, in which case the whole body is affected, and the mane and tail as well as hoofs are sometimes shed.

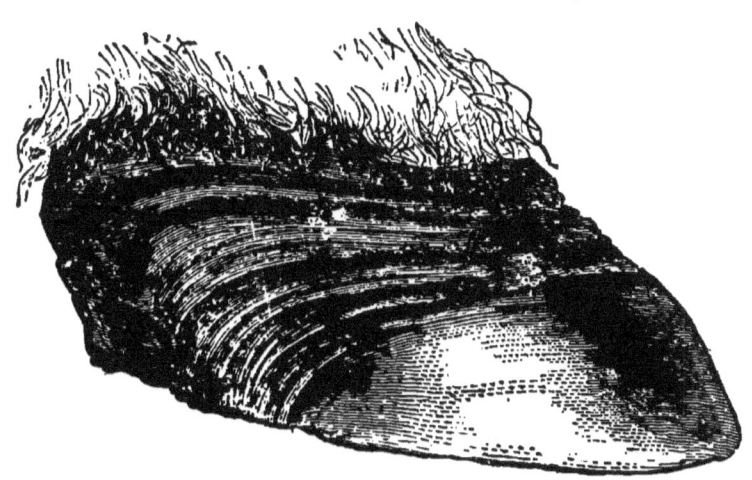

Fig. 83. Founder.

Remedy.—Remove shoes. Thin horn. Bed box with several inches of chaff or cut straw. Foment or poultice, hot; cold bran poultice over entire foot sometimes better than hot. Bleed from jugular or toe if severe, especially if caused by concussion. Repeated small doses of aconite, niter or other salines for fever. Half dose physic and laxative injections if needed. Vapor bath often serviceable. When inflammation is subdued, removal of exudate is hastened by cold applications; later by blisters to coronet; occasionally by frog setons. Keep heels low, toes short. Stout, wide-webbed, long-barred shoes.

If convexity and weakness of the sole result ('Pumiced Foot'), use bar shoe with wide web. Lessen concussion by tar dressing and leather soles. Stimulate coronet.

For doses, see pages 13 to 29.

MALLENDERS AND SALLENDERS

Are forms of psoriasis (scaly itch), which see. They are situated on the flexures of the knee and hock, that is, mallenders appear on the back of the knee, sallenders on the front of the hock. At first they are only scurfy patches, but exhibiting considerable irritability. If neglected, they degenerate into troublesome sores, with foul discharges.

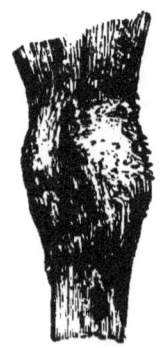
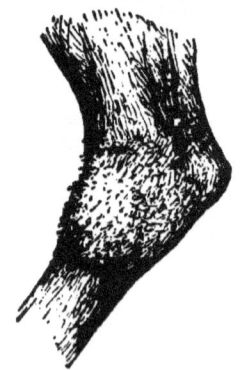

Fig. 84.   Mallenders.   Fig. 85.   Sallenders.

Remedy.—Soft soap and water, mild oils and bran poultices remove scales. Boro-glycerine or zinc oxide ointment. Mercuric nitrate or iodine ointments for thickening and infiltration. Tar oils for chronic cases. Half a dose of physic; salines; laxative diet. Iron tonics and arsenic for feeble. For doses, see pages 13 to 29.

RINGBONE

Is a bony tumor or bony deposit around the pastern joint or coffin joint, or both. It is of two kinds—true and false. The latter, as a rule, is almost harmless. True

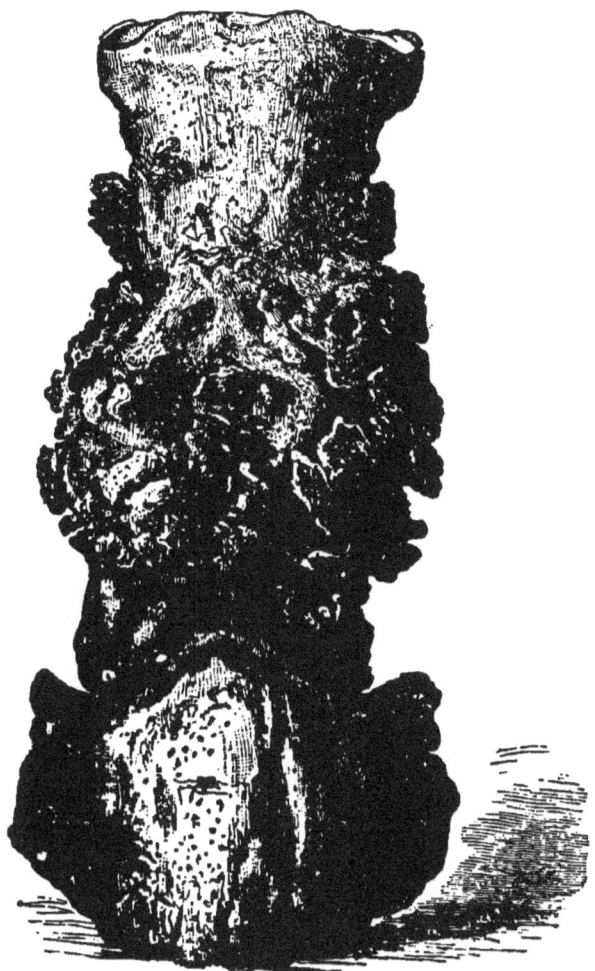

Fig. 86. High Ringbone.

ringbone is of two kinds—high and low. They are not the cause but the result of disease, especially inflammation of the bones and synovial membranes.

SIDEBONE

Is ossification of the lateral cartilages of the foot, usually the fore foot. Its causes are hereditary tendency and shoeing with high calkins.

Remedy.—Bar shoe; cold applications. Rest, blisters, firing, neurotomy (dissection and also section of a nerve).

SPRAIN OF THE BACK SINEWS

Of the hind legs is common among draft horses, especially those that are worked on hilly roads. The heel is hightened, and the first remedy is high calkins (Fig. 87). If the horse is worked, the foot and leg assume the position represented in Fig. 88.

When a horse's heel hightens, examine the back sinews. Feel them gently to discover if one place is tenderer, harder, or even slightly warmer than another. If this

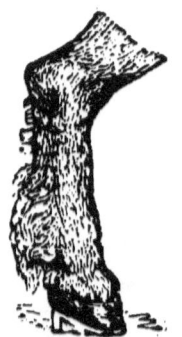

Fig. 87. High calkins for Sprain of the Back Sinews.

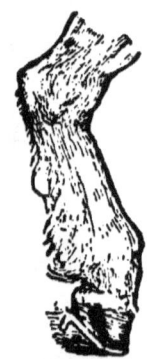

Fig. 88. The result of work after the sprain.

fails, pinch them hard and run the fingers down them, marking the part that causes flinching. Healthy tendon will endure any amount of pressure; diseased tendon is acutely sensitive. Cut the hair short and keep the part constantly damp with a linen bandage. Do not blister, bleed, seton, or fire. It requires from three to six months to effect a cure. The only remedy for a badly contracted tendon is its division, but the operation weakens the part.

WINDGALLS

Are soft swellings of the fetlock joints, formerly supposed to contain air. They really contain joint oil. They are sometimes as large as walnuts.

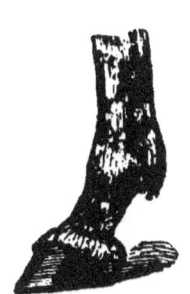 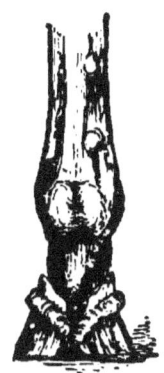

Fig. 89. Windgalls, before dissection.   Fig. 90.   After dissection.

Remedy.—Equable pressure by flannel or wash leather bandages. Bandages wetted with white lotion (¾ ounce of zinc sulphate, 1 ounce lead acetate, in quart of water). Rest, hand rubbing, blisters. Shoe so as to prevent concussion.

SEEDY TOE

Consists in the formation of a cheesy or mealy and therefore imperfect horn, which is incapable of maintaining the union between the outer wall and laminæ. When the defective horn shrinks, a crack is left for the reception of dirt. When not caused by inflammation or pressure of the shoe clip, it originates in some inherent cause, such as weak feet, &c. Lameness is not invariably present.

Remedy.—Remove diseased parts; promote growth of healthy horn by blisters and moisture. Bar shoes; sole pressure; remove shoe clips.

NAVICULAR DISEASE (Grogginess),

Is a rarifying inflammation of the navicular bone, with death of the articular cartilages and surrounding structures. The tendon of the flexor pedis perforans muscle is subsequently inflamed and becomes adherent to the navicular bone. Concussion and rheumatic predisposition are believed to be the chief causes. (Dun.)

It is the most fertile cause of lameness, and is the bane of horse flesh. Strain or laceration of the tendon is never a primary condition. The disease begins as an inflamma-

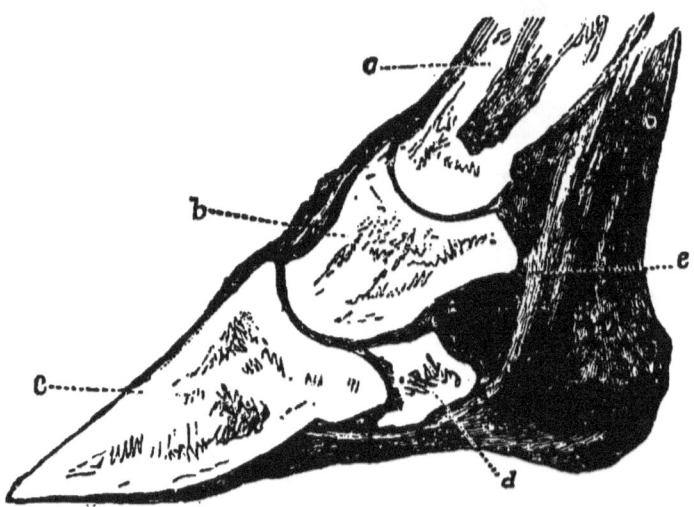

Fig. 91 represents the phalangeal bones in their naturally oblique position. The upper part of the long pastern bone (a), to toe of os pedis (c), is a continuously oblique line. This obliquity of position enables the bone to act as a spring, modifying concussion and giving elasticity of step and freedom from jar. The coronary bone (b) rests entirely on the os pedis. The navicular bone (d), placed posteriorly, bears no weight, but gives increased leverage power to the tendon (e). This bone, like the sesamoids, is a muscular appendage, and is not intended to support weight.
Compare with Fig. 92 on opposite page.

tion of the cancellated structure of the navicular bone, or of the cartilage on its inferior surface. It is caused by the rheumatoid diathesis (taint), concussion, and change in the relative position of the navicular bones, brought about by turned down, calkined, or thick heeled shoes. (Williams.)

Remedy.—Remove shoes and allow frog to come to the ground. Stand in cold water or apply cold wet swabs for several hours daily. Poultice at night. Physic and

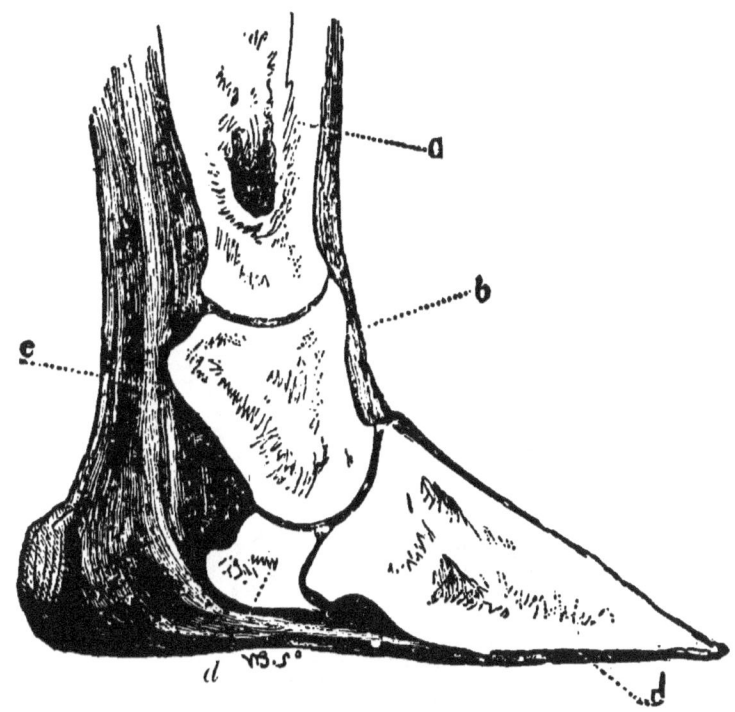

Fig. 92 represents the bones after their naturally oblique position has been changed to an almost perpendicular position by thick heeled shoes. The lower end of the os coronæ (*b*) rests partly on the navicular (*d*), instead of wholly on the pedal bone (*c*); hence the disease.

cooling diet. After 2 or 3 weeks blister coronet lightly. If necessary seton frog for 3 or 4 weeks. If disease still persists, relegate to slow work; shoes without heels or toe piece, or try neurotomy. Concussion is diminished by shoeing with leather and using shoes thick in quarters and thin at toe and heels.

HORN TUMOR (KERATOMA),

Is caused either by pressure of the toe clip of the shoe, the clip having been hammered too tightly by the smith, or by the animal striking the toe against the ground. These tumors are analogous to corns in the human feet, and consist of an increased secretion of horn. They are peculiar to the hind feet, but they are not uncommon in the fore.

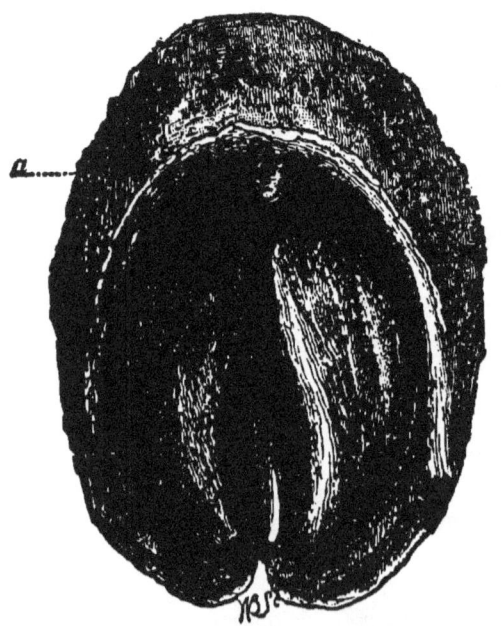

Fig. 93. Keratoma. *a*, horn tumor.

Remedy.—First try properly adjusted shoes. If this fails, isolate the diseased part by grooving, as in the process of 'stripping,' but leave the horn unstripped. Stripping consists in the removal of the whole of the crust immediately over the diseased part, by cutting through it on either side from top to bottom, detaching it from the sole, and tearing it off, leaving the sensitive parts exposed. This cruel treatment should never be resorted to

CAPPED HOCK

Is of two kinds—synovial and serous. The synovial appears as a tense, fluctuating swelling, on both sides of the point of the hock. It causes lameness and sometimes abscesses from caries of the bone. The serous (a watery abscess) is caused by pressure or violence, especially kicking. It is unsightly when large. It sometimes causes lameness.

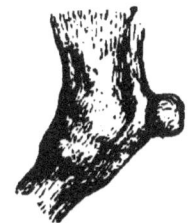
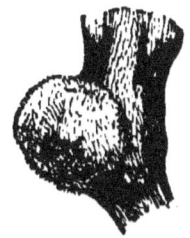

Fig. 94. Capped Hock.   Fig. 95. Large specimen of same.

Remedy.—Hot fomentations; then stimulate by cantharides liniment or mercuric iodide ointment; soft soap rubbed in daily. Equable pressure sometimes applied by truss. Evacuate serous abscess; inject cavity with iodine or astringents. In bursal form of capped hock use shoe raised at heel.

Treat **Capped Knee** and **Capped Elbow** the same as Capped Hock.

SANDCRACK

Consists of a fissure of greater or less extent in any part of the foot, but usually in the inner quarters of the fore and the toes of the hind feet. The crack opens and closes at every step, causing great pain and sometimes bleeding. Some horses seem to be predisposed to the disorder, but the cause is usually bad shoeing. Sandcrack never unites. A new crust must be cultivated.

Remedy.—Remove shoe, bottom crack, clear away dirt, and allow pus, if any, to escape. Foment, poultice, rest. Laxative when there is much pain and lameness. When these are abated, pare away upper part of cracked horn, cutting off connection with secreting coronary substance. Bar shoe, made to relieve cracked horn from pressure and concussion. When work is resumed, plug the crack with gutta-percha to keep out dirt. Hold split parts together by clasp, or by nails driven on the sides, with wire wrapped tightly around them. 'Stripping' in extreme cases only.

PUMICE FOOT

Is a deformity caused by hard work. A horse reared on marshy land usually has weak feet, which are soon deformed if it is worked on stony roads or streets. The symptoms are bulging sole, weak crust, strong bars, and good frog. The hoof is marked by rings, the pastern being long and slanting. (Mayhew). Dun says the disorder is caused by laminitis (described on page 201).

Remedy.—Bar shoe of the dish kind, with wide web. Leather soles to lessen concussion. Stimulate coronet.

SHIVERING OR JINKBACK

Is imperfect motor power or weakness of the back and loins, and is usually shown in backing or turning a horse rapidly. The forward movement may be natural. It is probably caused by disease of the spinal cord, but it may possibly sometimes be hereditary.

Remedy.—Treatment is of little avail. Light work without weight on back. Sling at night (for rest) if necessary.

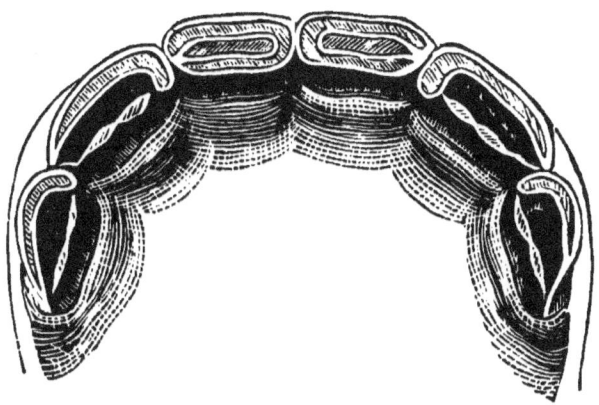

1-Year-Old, Lower Jaw (*Brandt*).

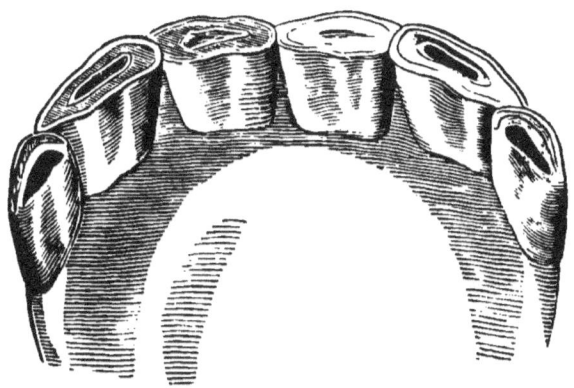

2-Year-Old, Lower Jaw; drawn from Nature.

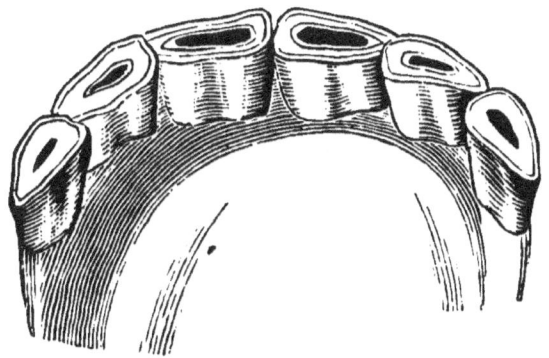

3-Year-Old, Lower Jaw; drawn from Nature.

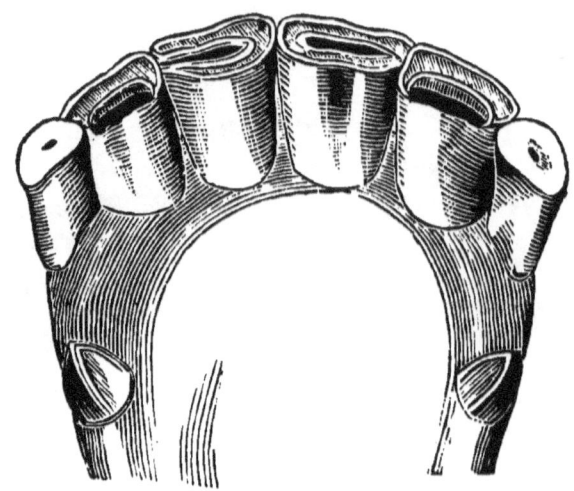

4-Year-Old, Lower Jaw; drawn from Nature.

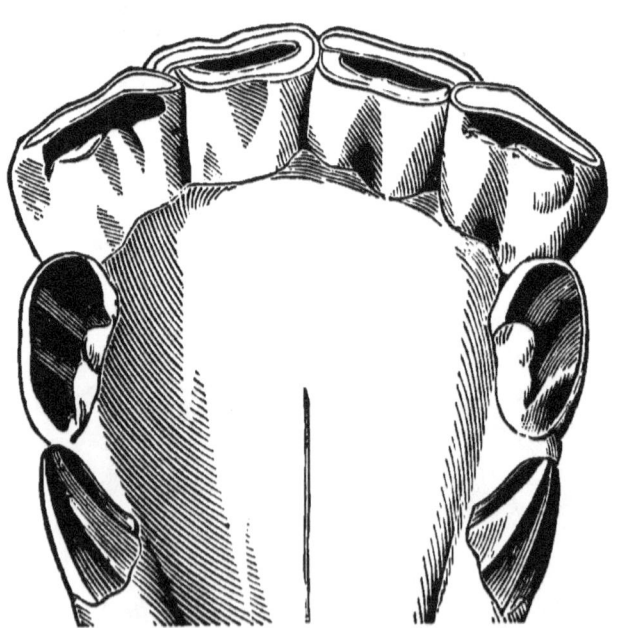

5-Year-Old, Lower Jaw; drawn from Nature.

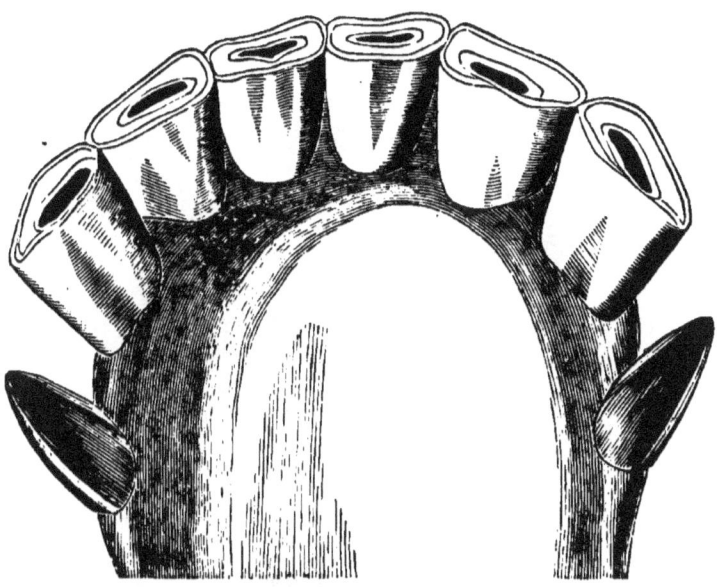

6-Year-Old, Lower Jaw; drawn from Nature.

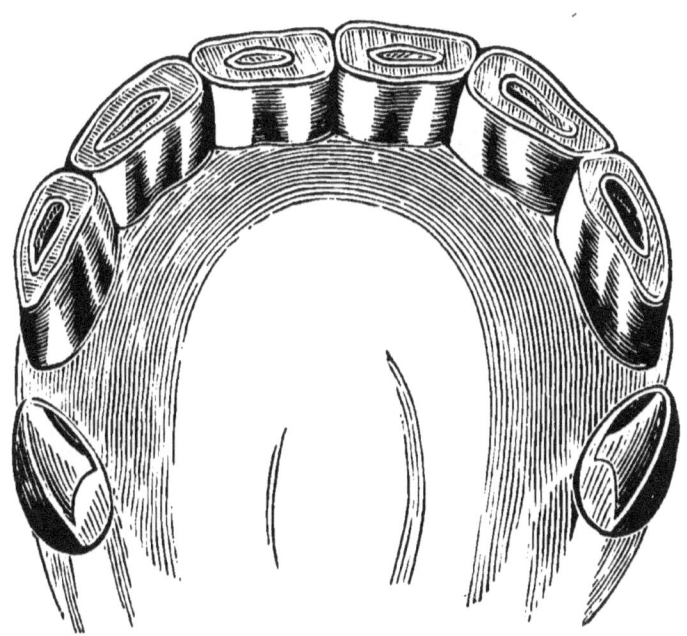

7-Year-Old, Lower Jaw (*Brandt*).

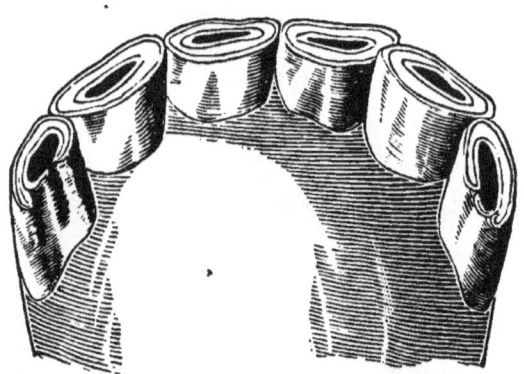

8-Year-Old, Upper Jaw (*Walsh*). About ⅔ nat. size.

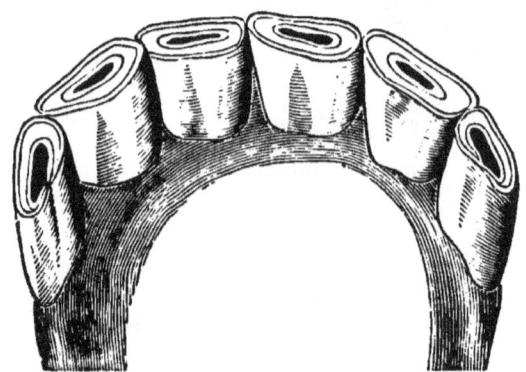

9-Year-Old, Upper Jaw (*Walsh*). About ⅔ nat. size.

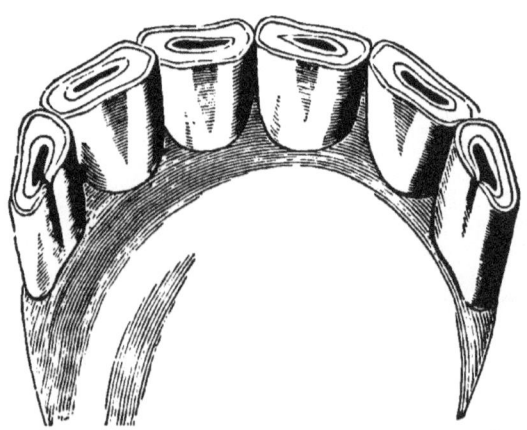

10-Year-Old, Upper Jaw (*Walsh*). About ⅔ nat. size.

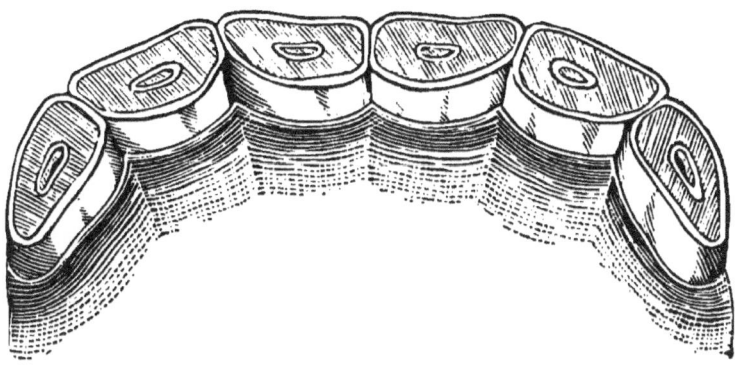

11 years, Upper Jaw. The marks have disappeared.

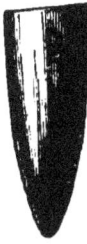

The Mark, dissected as it were. (See page 221.)

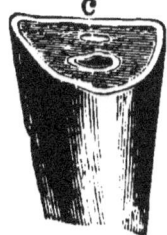

c, The Dentinal star, sometimes mistaken for the mark. (See page 221.)

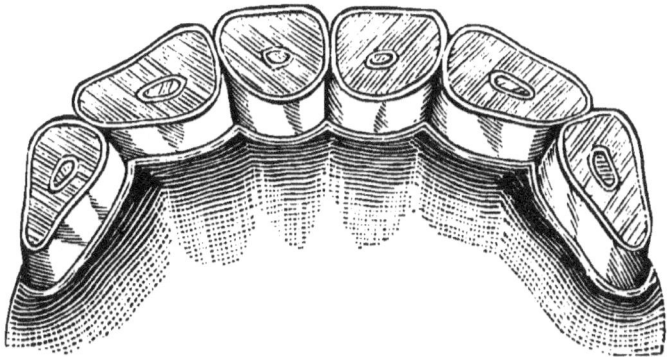

12 years, Lower Jaw. Change in shape is now clearly defined. The respective pairs (centrals, dividers, corners) assume in turn (from 12 years till old age) various shapes—semi-square, rounded, triangular, wedge-shaped, etc.

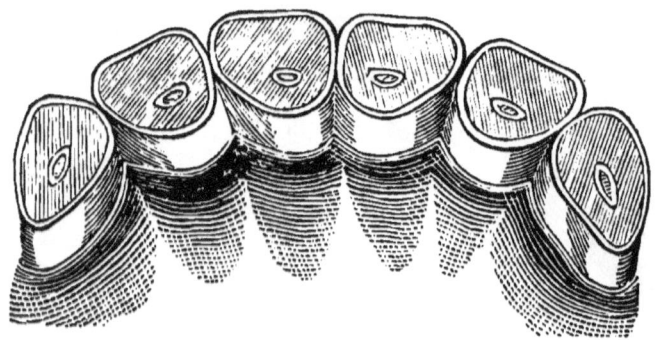

13 years, Lower Jaw.

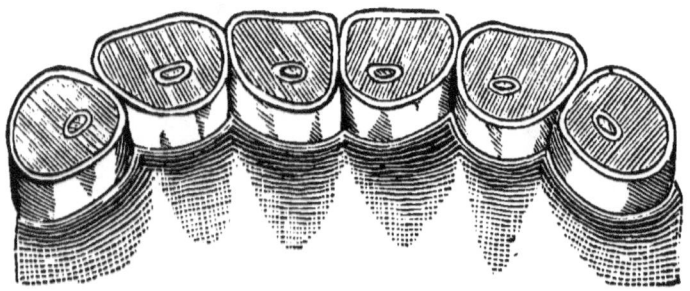

14 years, Lower Jaw.

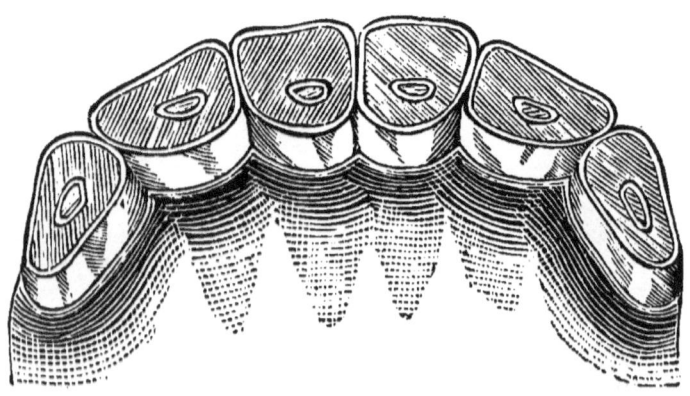

15 years, Upper Jaw.

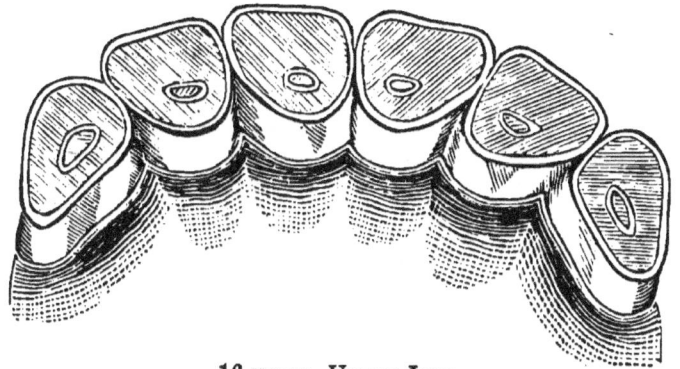

16 years, Upper Jaw.

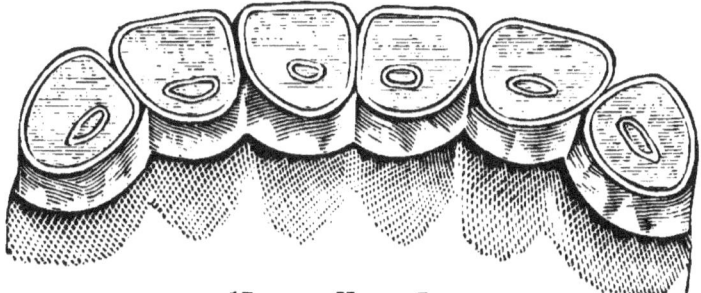

17 years, Upper Jaw.

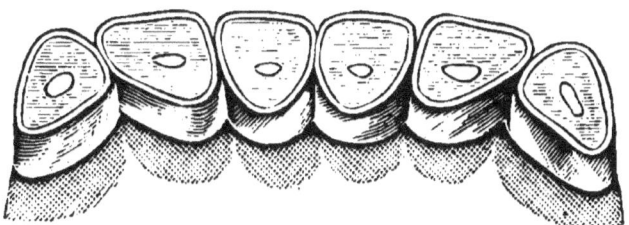

18 years, Lower Jaw.

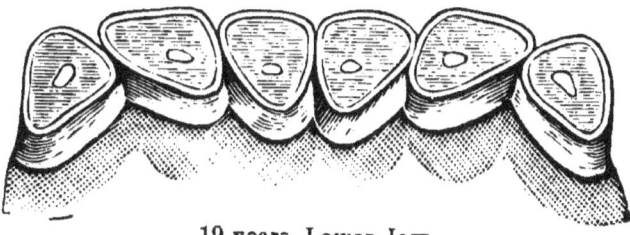

19 years, Lower Jaw.

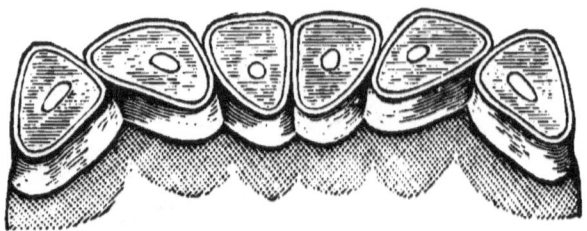

20 years, Lower Jaw.

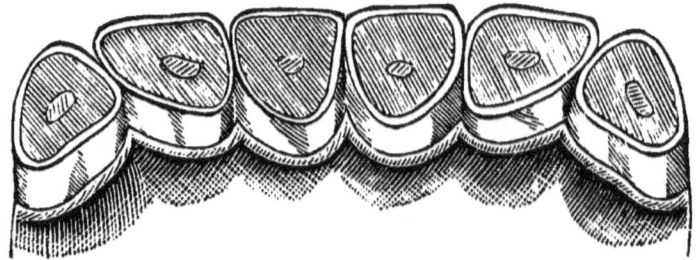

21 years, Upper Jaw.

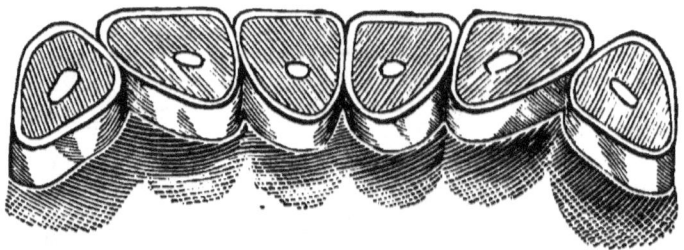

22 years, Upper Jaw.

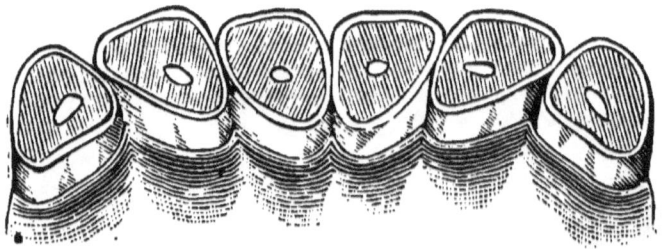

23 years, Upper Jaw.

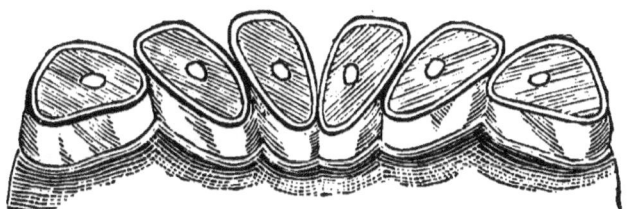

24 years, Lower Jaw.

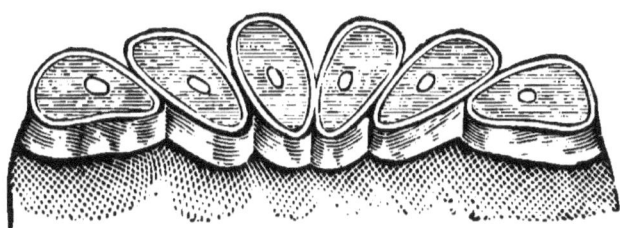

25 years, Lower Jaw.

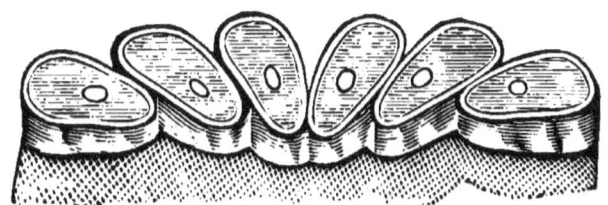

26 years, Lower Jaw.

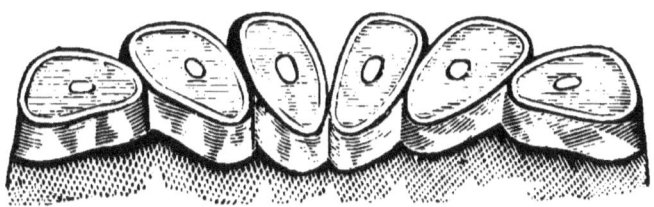

27 years, Upper Jaw.

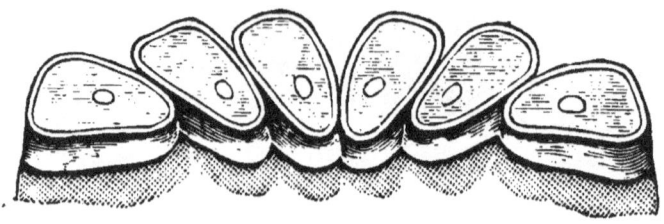

28 years, Upper Jaw.

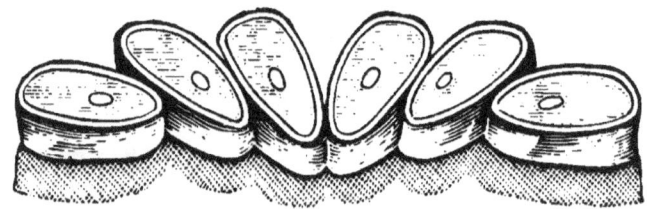

29 years, Upper Jaw.

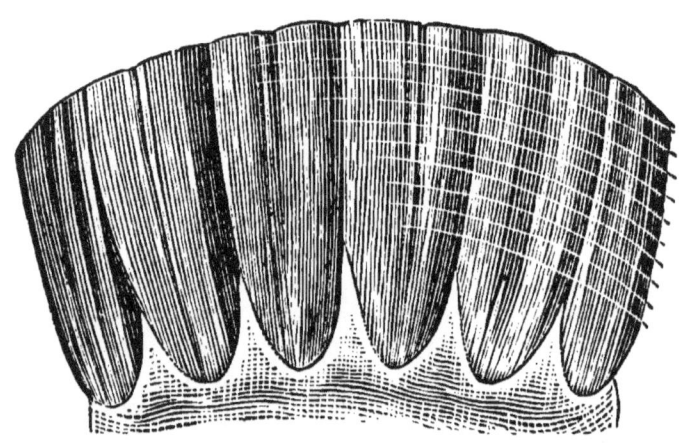

A Parrot-Mouth (lower jaw). The ten lines represent ten years' growth. The marks, having never been worn, represent a 6-year-old. The horse is therefore 16 years old. (This cut, as well as many of the preceding, is from Braudt's "Age of Horses.")

THE MARK AND DENTINAL STAR.

(Illustrated on page 215.)

The mark (also called central enamel, infundibulum, &c.) is composed of enamel, the hardest of the three constituent parts of the teeth—enamel, dentine, and cement.

The dentinal star, so called because it is composed of dentine, appears about the ninth year. It has a yellow tint, which is the best means of distinguishing it from the mark. Its appearance is accounted for as follows: When the tooth wears nearly to the pulp or nerve cavity, the pulp becomes gradually converted into dentine, filling the upper part of the cavity from the inside as perfectly as a dentist can fill a cavity from the outside. The star is visible eight or ten years. After it is worn out, there will be a cavity of course.

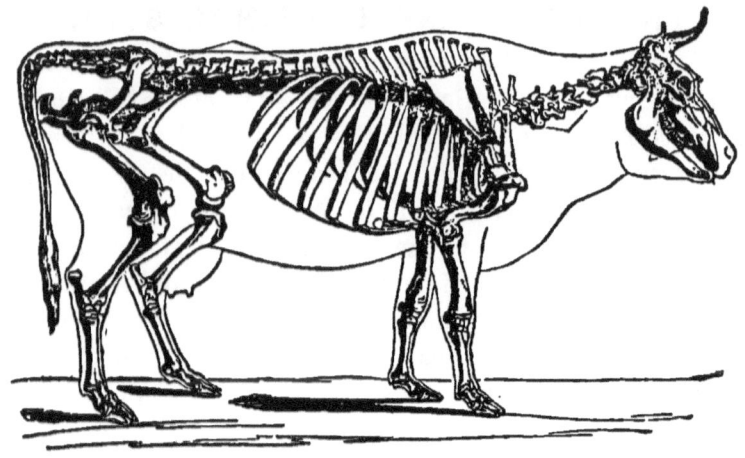

Fig. 96. Skeleton of Cow.

PART II.

THE DISEASES OF CATTLE.

CONTAGIOUS PLEURO-PNEUMONIA,

Also called lung disease, pulmonary murrain, zymotic or epizootic pleuro-pneumonia, &c., is an incurable febrile disease. Gresswell says it is believed to be generated by and due to a definite micrococcus (mite). It may be acute, subacute, or chronic.

Symptoms.—Elevation of temperature or a slight cough is usually the first sign. The temperature will range from 100 to 107°. Shiverings; hair stands wrong way; slight loss of appetite; breathing difficult and laborious; nostrils dilated; flanks heave; mouth hot; muzzle dry; gums pale, lilac color; walls of chest, rib spaces, and back from withers to loins more or less sensitive to pressure; appetite worse; milk diminishes; emaciation begins; bowels irregular; watery or sticky discharge from nostrils; abnormal sounds in bronchial tubes and mucous rattle over lungs; cough worse; back arched and head and neck extended when coughing.

In what is called the second stage, these symptoms are intensified and others appear: Death sometimes occurs in the first stage.

Remedy.—Slaughter and general and thorough disinfection of premises. Vaccination and inoculation should be left to the veterinarian.

'Sporadic Pleuro-Pneumonia' is described by Gresswell. He says it is "amenable to judicious treatment."

FOOT AND MOUTH DISEASE,

Also called eczema contagiosa, eczema epizootica, epizootic aphtha, aphthous fever, murrain, epidemic, &c., is a highly contagious and infectious febrile disease, associated with a vesicular eruption in the mouth, between the pedal digits, and around the coronets. In some cases the mouth only is affected; in others the feet only. In milk cows the mammary glands and lactiferous ducts are sometimes affected. When this is the case, the milk is unfit for use for either man or beast, for it may cause eruptions in the mouth, larynx, pharynx, and alimentary canal. Sheep, goats, swine, dogs, poultry, and even human beings are liable to the disease.

Dr. Klein says the disease is due to micrococci (mites). Mild cases require little treatment, as the disease runs a definite course and ends in recovery in about a week.

Remedy.—Salicylate sodium, 3 drams, spirit nitrous ether, 1 fluid oz., water, 7 oz., twice daily.

Sulphite sodium, 3 drams, water 8 oz., 2 or 3 times daily.

Sulphite sodium, 3 drams, aniseeds, 1 oz., fenugreek, 1 oz., in food 3 times daily, when other medicines are not given.

Gargles: 1. Boric acid, 1 part, glycerine, 5 fluid parts, water, 11 parts, several times daily. 2. Acid solution nitrate mercury, 4 drops, water, 1 oz., several times daily. 3. Permanganate potassium, 3 to 4 grains, water, 1 oz., 2 or 3 times daily.

Ointments for feet and teats: 1. Boric acid, 1 part, vaselin, 3 parts, lard, 3 parts. 2. Carbolic acid, 1 part, lard or vaselin, 30 parts. 3. Iodoform, 20 grains, oil eucalyptus, 20 drops, carbolic acid, 20 drops, lard or vaselin, 1½ oz. Latter especially good for sores and ulcers.

TUBERCULAR CONSUMPTION (TUBERCULOSIS),

Which is so prevalent among cattle, is doubtless caused by a bacillus (atmospheric mite). It may be found, says Gresswell, that bovine tuberculosis can be stamped out as cattle plague, foot and mouth disease, sheep scab, pleuro-pneumonia, and rabies can. There are indications that protective inoculation with tubercular matter obtained from fowl which have died of the disease will throw light on a method of prevention.

Symptoms.—In well developed cases the ox is emaciated; sluggish movements; dull look; eyes sunken; skin dry and adheres to ribs; hair lacks healthy luster and is often damp; slight exertion causes sweating, laborious breathing, and great distress; great weakness, sometimes even lowering the head to the ground for relief; membranes of mouth and other orifices pale yellow; appetite capricious and less than in health; dejections (excrements) bad; stomach may be more or less distended with gas; constipation and diarrhea may alternate; coughs up a viscid, usually inodorous, but sometimes offensive matter, which may contain yellowish cheesy flakes, &c.

Remedy.—Well developed cases are incurable. In mild attacks fatten and slaughter. In milk cows, stop milking; give fattening food, such as oil cake and good hay; avoid grasses and roots. If there are any ulcerating scrofulous glands, dress with carbolic acid and chalk or some other antiseptic.

CARBUNCULAR FEVER (ANTHRAX),

Also called Texas fever, splenic fever, trembles, charbon, blain, &c., is supposed to be the disease referred to in Exodus, chapter ix, as the "boil which came forth as blains upon man and beast throughout all Egypt." (Robertson.)

The disease is contagious, very rapid in its course, and is caused by the vegetable organism bacillus anthracis. It is both enzootic and epizootic, occurring whenever and wherever conditions favor the growth of the germs, one of which is rainy weather followed by heat.

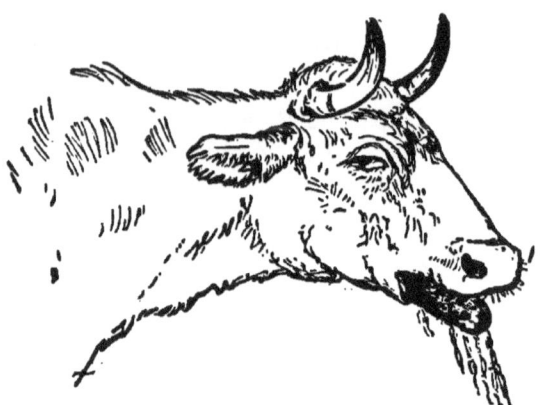

Fig. 97. Gloss-Anthrax or Blain, early stage.

Symptoms.—Stops feeding and chewing cud suddenly; shivers; moves stiffly and unsteadily; limbs rigid; soon falls and is unable to move; may, however, stand for a while, back curved. The spleen is usually especially affected, but sometimes it is the bowels; severe convulsions are not uncommon; tenacious mucus flows from mouth; tongue becomes of a darker hue; belly distended; passes liquid and blood-stained excreta and sometimes a large quantity of dark blood; blood sometimes flows from nostrils; white of eyes become dark red; eyes sink in orbit; tears flow over face, &c.

Death may follow in a few minutes, hours, or a day. Recovery is rare.

Remedy.—Sulphite sodium, 3 drams, salicylate sodium, 3 drams, tincture aconite (B. P.), 40 drops, water a sufficient quantity, every 4 hours.

Liquified carbolic acid, 30 drops, gentian, 2 oz., aniseed, 2 oz., in pint of water every 4 hours.

GENERAL DISEASES.

Mix 12 oz. (ounces) each of carbolic acid and sodium bicarbonate with 4 fluid oz. of glycerine; give 2 tablespoonfuls of the mixture in a quart of water 3 times daily. The latter mixture is much used in America.

Kill all hopelessly sick cattle and bury the carcasses 6 feet deep, spreading quick lime over them. Disinfect premises and everything used in treating the sick. Separate sick from well.

BLACK-LEG OR BLACK QUARTER,

Also called symptomatic anthrax, quarter ill, inflammatory fever, carbuncular erysipelas, emphysema infectuosum, speed, Chabert's disease, &c., is a very fatal and infectious disease. It is caused by a rod-like germ very similar to the 'bacillus anthracis.'

The disease is peculiar to calves and cattle under two years of age. Setoning the dew-lap (fold of skin on throat), first dressing the seton with black oil, is said to be an almost certain preventive. Recovery from this disease is rare. Death usually occurs in two or three days from blood poisoning.

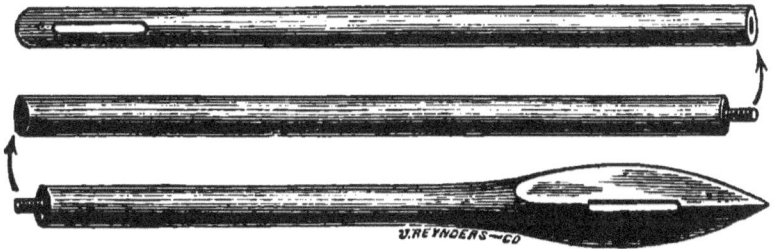

Fig. 98. Three-jointed, sharp Seton Needle.

Symptoms.—Dull; listless; lame in one or two limbs, either hind or fore; appetite fails; stops chewing cud; thirst; head protruded; white of eye bloodshot; mouth hot; moans; if forced to move, staggers and drops down; constipated; then feces become soft and tinged with blood; skin dry and rough; harsh and staring coat; urine, at first high colored, becomes deeply blood stained; loins, back, ribs tender; painful swellings at fetlock, knee joint, hock joint, stifle, elbow, or shoulder, which may soon mortify, &c.

Remedy.—Gentle laxative, then sulphite sodium, 1 dram, salicylate sodium, 1 dram, water a sufficient quantity, every 6 hours.

Incise and dress tumors, if large, with carbolic acid, 1 part, water, 25. Good hay, mashes, linseed, or oatmeal gruel. Drain wet pastures.

CATTLE PLAGUE

Is a contagious febrile disease, and is probably caused by a micrococcus. It is peculiar to Asia.

ACTINOMYCOSIS,

Known in the past as cancerous, scrofulous, or schirrous tongue, in Germany as wooden tongue and throat boil, is characterized by tumors of various size and shape on the tongue, jaw, tooth sockets, bones, and soft tissues of the head, from which parts it may spread. It is described as "a new and infectious disease of animals and man." In cattle it is due to a fungus called 'actinomyces' (ray fungus). Moldy straw, barley, or chaff, especially if the mouth be sore or lacerated, is liable to cause the disease. Moldy foods usually contain vegetable parasites. As in foot and mouth disease, an ox will slaver and champ and chew its hay, but will usually eject it. But it will eat mashes and linseed gruel.

Remedy.—Incise the tumors and then apply the following mixture: Iodine, 1 part, carbolic acid, 4 fluid parts, glycerine, 4 fluid parts. Tincture of iodine, plain or diluted with alcohol (methylated or not), will answer.

Gargle: Acid solution nitrate mercury, 8 drops, water, 1 oz. Will do for wash also after incision of tumors.

Tonics if necessary. Soft, nutritious food.

RABIES OR HYDROPHOBIA.

(See page 50.)

COW-POX VARIOLA VACCINÆ),

Affects the udder and teats of cows chiefly. The rash consists of small, pale red, hard pustules, varying in size from a pea to a horse-bean. The pustules are converted into vesicles containing a viscid, yellow fluid. These gradually increase in size, until in about eight and a half days they are about five-eighths of an inch in diameter. In the center they have a light blue tint, but toward the margin they are reddish blue or yellow. Their contents now become purulent. The center is usually depressed, and a crust begins to form there, gradually extending to the periphery. The border is hard, swollen, and painful and a red areola forms, together with much thickening under the skin.

About the fourteenth day a scab, which is thick, dark, adherent, and shining, is formed, and about the fifteenth day it becomes detatched, having a depressed scar, which is at first bluish red, but gradually turns pale, and persists for a long time.

The febrile symptoms are very slight and usually unimportant. The infection is not dangerous. A partial loss of appetite, an abstention from chewing the cud, trifling constipation, diminution, and deterioration of the milk are observable. The udder is swollen, especially near the teats, and milking causes pain. There may be more than one eruption of pustules.

The disease usually lasts about seventeen and a half days, but may be protracted to about five weeks, during which time the milk is unfit for use.

Remedy.—Give a laxative and draw off milk with a siphon. Draft: Solution acetate ammonium, 4 fluid oz., tincture aconite (V. P.), 40 drops, water a sufficient quantity, 3 times daily.

DIPHTHERIA,

Or a disease resembling it, sometimes affects cattle.

Symptoms.—Throat sore and swollen; coughing spells; flow of saliva from mouth and mucus from nostrils; accelerated breathing, causing a crowing sound during inspiration; may be spasms of larynx, especially if animal is excited; great debility finally supervenes; pulse, at first quick, grows weaker and weaker as the disease progresses; cough worse; about the third day lymph-casts of parts of the air tubes, or flakes of lymph at least, are ejected.

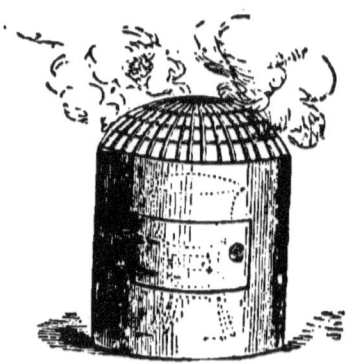

Fig. 99. Steaming apparatus for Diphtheria, Catarrh, Bronchitis, &c. See Fig. 100, an equally good and simpler method.

Remedy.—Careful nursing. Liquid food. Steam air passages with an antiseptic inhalation, such as about a teaspoonful of oil of eucalyptus to about a gallon of boiling water; a free supply of water containing about a dram of chlorate of potassium to half bucket water. Good air. Salicylic acid, 1 dram, is useful; also same quantity sulphite sodium.

Puncture throat if there is danger of suffocation. Tonics if necessary.

MALIGNANT CATARRH,

A very fatal disease, causing death in from three to seven days, is said to be non-contagious and to result from inflammation induced by exposure to cold. (See 'Catarrh,' the simple form, page, 70.)

Symptoms.—Shivering fits; dull look; membranes bluish red; eyes close; eyelids swell; tears flow over cheeks; painful, frequent cough; feeble pulse; constipation followed by diarrhea; profuse discharges from nostrils and mouth; sometimes the horns drop off.

Remedy.—Remove to warm sheds. Tincture perchloride of iron, 1 fluid oz., salicine, 1 dram, simple sirup, 4 fluid oz., water a sufficient quantity, 3 times daily.

Gargle: Acid solution nitrate mercury, 6 drops, water, 1 oz.; or, permanganate potassium, 3 to 4 grains, water, 1 oz.

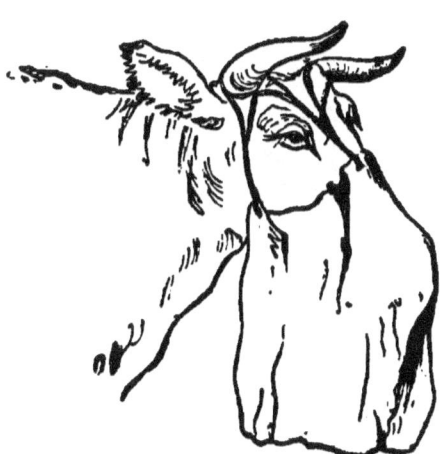

Fig. 100. Steam-bag for Catarrh.

Purge if necessary. Inhale steam from boiling water, in which put a small portion of oil of eucalyptus or carbolic acid, as above for diphtheria. Tonics and good food during convalescence.

RHEUMATISM,

Like tetanus (lock-jaw), is practically the same in the ox as in the horse. (See page 63.)

Remedy.—Tincture aconite (V. P.), 30 drops, salicylate sodium, 4 drams, bicarbonate potassium, 1 oz., water in proportion, every 6 hours. Or, tincture colchicum, $\frac{1}{2}$

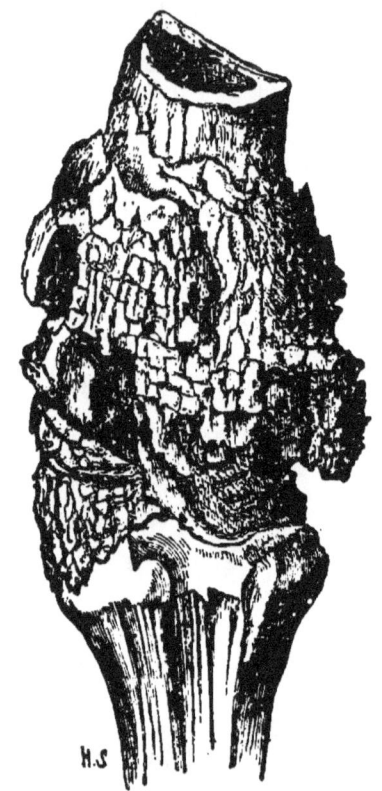

Fig. 101. Knee joint after Chronic Rheumatism.

oz., tincture aconite (V. P.), 30 drops, bicarbonate potassium, 1 oz., water in proportion, every 6 hours.

Liniment: Alcohol, 1 pint, ammonia, $\frac{1}{2}$ oz., oil organum, $\frac{1}{2}$ oz., oil sassafras, $\frac{1}{2}$ oz., tincture capsicum, $\frac{1}{2}$ oz., tincture opium, $\frac{1}{2}$ oz., spirit turpentine, $\frac{1}{2}$ oz., camphor, $\frac{1}{4}$ oz.

RICKETS OR RACHITIS (Bone Softening),

When not hereditary, is caused by a lack of health-giving food. It is peculiar to young animals. Give 1½ to 3 drams phosphate of lime once a day, or cod liver oil, 4 oz., lime water, 2 oz., once a day. Nutritious diet and pure air. (See page 69.)

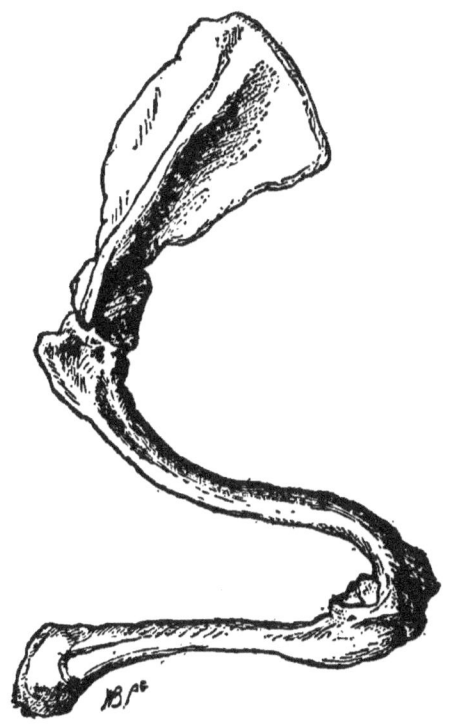

Fig. 102. Rickets in humerus of dog.

BONE BRITTLENESS (FRAGILITAS OSSIUM),

Is rare except in districts where the water and soil are lacking in lime salts and phosphates. The general health is affected and fractures are common.

Remedy.—Change pasture and water and feed on nutritious, phosphatic foods. The salts of iron are valuable tonics. Sulphate or carbonate of iron is useful, but the citrate of iron and ammonium, in 2-dram doses, twice a day, is even better. Vegetable tonics and the phosphate of calcium are valuable. Soft water seems to be bad for cows. (See 'Osteoporosis,' page 68.

ANÆMIA (Lack of Blood),

Is caused by underfeeding or unhealthy food. Prevent by good feeding, and if medicine is necessary, give any of the following:

Powdered gentian, 1½ oz., powdered ginger, ½ oz., granulated sulphate of iron, 2 drams, powdered nux vomica, 40 grains, powdered capsicum, ½ dram, in a pint of water, gruel, or ale, twice daily.

Powdered gentian, 1 oz., powdered ginger, ½ oz., carbonate ammonium, ½ oz., carbonate iron, 2 drams, in a pint of warm water, gruel, or ale, twice daily.

Solution hydrochlorate strychnine, 2 drams, tincture capsicum, 4 drams, tincture perchloride iron, 1 oz., in pint of warm water or gruel, once daily.

DIABETES,

Though rare, is practically the same in the ox as in the horse. (See page 63.) The remedies should be the same as for anæmia (above), giving a laxative first if necessary.

TETANUS (LOCK-JAW),

Is not as common in the ox as in the horse. If the jaws are not too firmly locked, give bromide potassium, 4 drams, anise fruit, 4 drams, in warm water or gruel, thrice daily. (See page 53.)

GOITER

Is enlargement of the thyroid gland, and is caused by water obtained from magnesian limestone. It may be hereditary. Change water, or use rain water or water acted on by carbonate of sodium. It is more common in sheep than cattle. (See page 78.)

SCARLET FEVER

Is a specific, contagious, and infectious disease, communicable perhaps even to man by means of the milk and inoculation. It is peculiar to recently calved cows. The disease lasts from five weeks to even three months. It is caused by a micrococcus.

Symptoms.—Short fever; quick breathing; hacking cough; sore throat in severe cases; discharges from nostrils and eyes; eruption on skin around eyes; also hind quarters; vesicles on teats and udder; teats double in size; vesicles, at first the size of a pea, enlarge to half-inch ulcers, with reddish brown scabs; scabs may remain 25 days or longer; watery fluid exudes from under scab; ulcers leave a whitish, flat, indistinct scar, &c.

Remedy.—Solution acetate ammonium, 4 fluid ounces; spirit nitrous ether, 1 fluid oz., bicarbonate potassium, $\frac{1}{2}$ oz., water, $3\frac{1}{2}$ oz., 3 times a day. Draw off milk with siphon. Feed calf by hand.

PURPLE FEVER (PURPURA HÆMORRHAGICA),

Is a specific, eruptive blood fever, of an intermittent type, in which the skin, mucous membranes, connective tissue of the lungs and kidneys and coats of the intestinal walls are mainly affected. It seems to result from exposure or foul air, and often follows a disease like catarrhal fever. It runs its course in about a week, and, like anthrax, which it resembles, is often fatal. It is peculiar to calves rather than adults. (See page 47.)

Symptoms.—Pain and slight swellings in one or more limbs; may be purple or dark red spots in nostrils and pimples on skin; blood seems to be thinner than usual; it or red serum, or both, exudes, especially on the mucous and serous membranes; temperature changeable, but may suddenly reach 106° F. or more; hot and rather circumscribed swellings appear on various parts of the body, from which, and also from the nostrils, a reddish fluid flows; these swellings interfere somewhat with breathing and swallowing; heart weak and fluttering; pulse small and double.

Remedy.—Nutritious, digestible food. Stimulants.

Drafts: 1. Quinetum (mixed alkaloids from cinchona bark), 1 dram, tincture perchloride iron, 1 fluid oz., oil turpentine, $\frac{1}{2}$ fluid oz., water in proportion, twice daily. 2. Powdered gentian, 1 oz., powdered ginger, $\frac{1}{2}$ oz., carbonate ammonium, $\frac{1}{2}$ oz., carbonate iron, 2 drams, in pint warm water, gruel, or ale, twice daily.

POISONS.

Among the poisonous plants and minerals common to cattle are the following:

Meadow Saffron or Autumn Crocus. Give mucilage of linseed with 2 ounces spirit ammonia and 4 ounces brandy every 4 hours.

Aconite. Give 2 ounces spirit ammonia with 4 ounces of brandy in gruel every 2 hours, repeated as often as necessary.

Yew. Give 4 ounces spirit of ammonia with 8 ounces brandy in quart of mucilage linseed, repeated in 1 hour, and at intervals of 2, 3, or 4 hours if necessary. Purge with 8 to 10 drams of aloes, followed by a quart of linseed oil after the first draft. Mustard to belly. Open paunch and remove foliage if necessary.

Woody Nightshade. Treat as for yew. It is often fatal.

Ergot is caused by the growth of a fungoid parasite which infests most of the grasses and cereals. It is most common in damp situations. Cut the grass when in full bloom, and thus prevent the formation of ergot. Tannin and stimulants are antidotes for ergot.

Arsenic. Copious quantities of linseed mucilage and gruel. Hydrated peroxide of iron, 1 ounce every hour for 3 or 4 hours; then every 3 hours for a day or so. Stimulate with spirit of ammonia and brandy and give tincture of opium in 2-ounce doses for pain if it is necessary.

Lead. Epsom salt, 10 ounces, Glauber's salt, 10 ounces, 4 drams diluted sulphuric acid, 20 drops croton oil, in gruel. Repeat in 8 or 10 hours, giving half the quantity only. After the first draft, mucilage of linseed or gruel should be given in large quantities every hour; and at each alternate hour 4 drams of diluted sulphuric acid may be added.

DISEASES OF THE ALIMENTARY SYSTEM.

THRUSH OR APHTHA

Is practically the same in cattle as in sheep. (See sheep.) As in the human species, young animals, especially sucking calves, are often attacked. The disease is usually mild unless the vesicles or tiny bladders extend to the gullet, stomach, or intestines.

Begin the treatment with a gentle aperient; then gargle with chlorate of potassium or alum, 15 grains to each ounce of water, 2 or 3 times daily. Laxative diet. In severe cases carbonate of ammonium and other stimulants are necessary.

HOVEN (TYMPANITES),

Also known as hove, hoove, blown, dew-blown, fog-sickness, &c., is an important and common disease in cattle and sheep, but is usually curable if taken in time

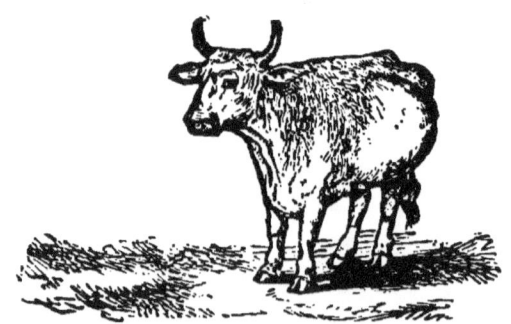

Fig. 103. Hoven.

and properly treated. The swelling, as is shown in the illustration, is on the left side.

The swelling is caused by gas in the first stomach (the rumen or paunch), and is usually the result of injudicious feeding. Sudden change from a poor diet to a rich one is bad, for it causes overeating. The swelling is sometimes chronic, when it may depend on the presence of foreign bodies in the rumen.

Remedy.—Begin with a purge; then give hyposulphite of sodium, ½ oz., water in proportion, and repeat several times at intervals of from 2 to 4 hours.

2. Ether, 2 fluid oz., carbonate ammonium, ½ oz., spirit chloroform, 1 fluid oz., water in proportion, at intervals of 4 hours.

3. Sulphocarbolate sodium, ½ oz., bromide potassium, 2 drams, chlorodyne, 6 fluid drams, water in proportion, at intervals of from 4 to 6 hours.

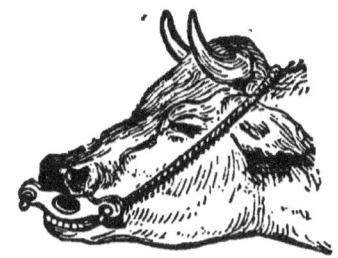

Fig. 104. Mode of securing ox in passing Probang for either gas or choking.

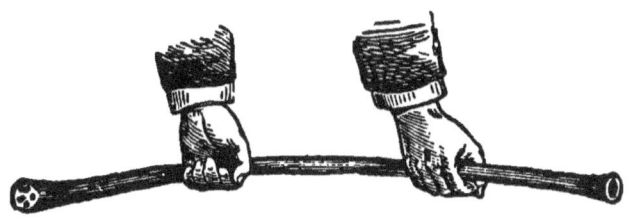

Fig. 105. The Probang.

When foreign substances or food causes choking, the use of the probang is necessary, provided the obstructing body cannot be reached with the hand. The probang should be 6 or 7 feet in length. Its use is illustrated in Figs. 104, 105. Some animals require to be very securely fastened, while others may be held by hand.

ENGORGEMENT OF THE OMASUM OR THIRD STOMACH (OMASITIS),

Also called fardel-bound and grass staggers, is probably caused by old fog-grass, straw, dry, harsh, and badly cured hay, and any coarse herbage or heath. Very bad hay can only be made slightly available by being mixed with a large quantity of cut turnips, mangold-wurzel, or grain.

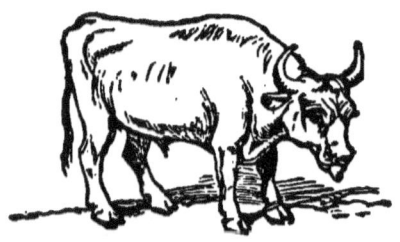

Fig. 106. Impaction of the Omasum.

Symptoms.—Head held low; ears hang; breathing difficult; tip of tongue protrudes; eyes staring and blood-shot; sight impaired; grunts and moans; grinds teeth; head pointed toward abdomen, usually the right side, on account of pain; hind legs often moved; tail lashed; rumen often swelled; staggers, rolls on side and lies there with rigid limbs; convulsions and death.

Remedy.—In ordinary cases Epsom salt, 16 oz. or more, clears the way for aloes, the former acting on the bowels, the latter on the stomach. Oil is useful as an adjunct. External stimulating for stomach inflammation. Give injections regularly, and watch animal carefully. Nitrated drinking water. Sulphate of physostygmine, dissolved, has been injected both intravenously and hypodermically (in the veins and under the skin) in doses of $\frac{1}{2}$ to $1\frac{1}{2}$ grain.

ENGORGEMENT AND INFLAMMATION OF THE RUMEN (PLENALVIA),

Which is caused by excessive quantities of food, entails more suffering than hoven, which is caused mostly by gas. The disorders are easily distinguished. The swelling in hoven resembles an inflated bladder and is resonant on percussion, while the engorged stomach has a soft, doughy feel and pits on pressure. The swelling is on the left side in both disorders. The animal is dull; suffers

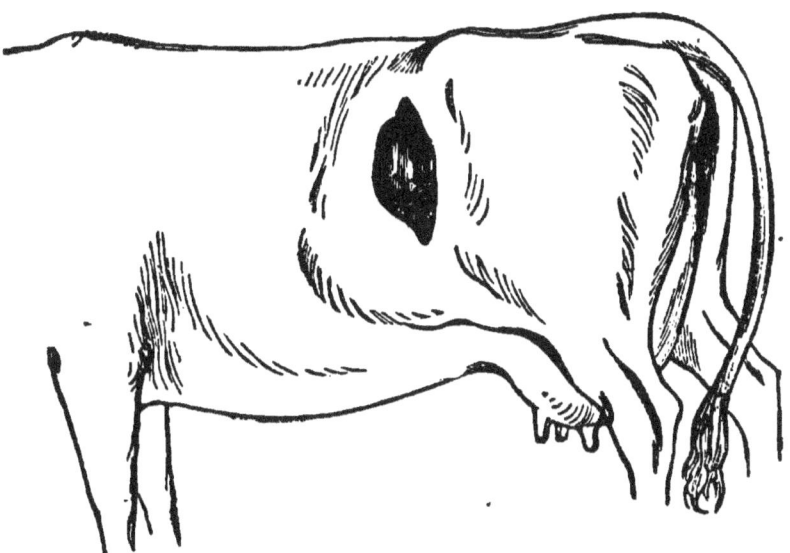

Fig. 107. The rumen exposed for mechanical removal of contents.

pain; no appetite; constipated, feces being hard and glazed; pulse small and quick; lies on right side. Hoven usually follows, accompanied by difficult breathing, moaning, grinding teeth, arching back, protruding muzzle, &c.

Sometimes the paunch is opened and its contents removed by hand, but this operation should be performed by the veterinarian only. (Fig. 107.)

The rumen is sometimes ruptured in both hoven and

engorgement, and is usually soon followed by death. Hair balls, caused by cattle licking themselves or one another, and calculous concretions sometimes form in the rumen, reticulum, and abomasum (the first, second, and fourth of the four stomachs). See page 111 for 'Calculous Concretions.'

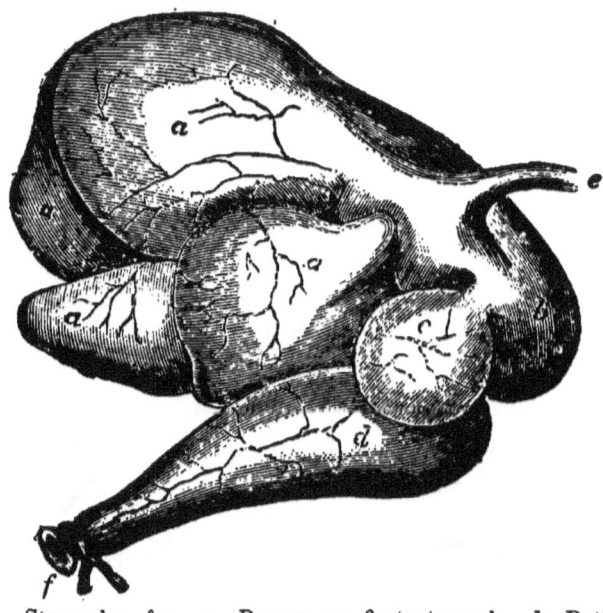

Fig. 108. Stomachs, &c. $a_{1.}$ Rumen or first stomach. b, Reticulum or second stomach. c, Omasum or third stomach. d, Abomasum or fourth stomach. e, Esophagus, throat or gullet. f, Pylorus, entrance to intestines.

Remedy.—Epsom salt, 16 oz., solution of aloes, 4 to 8 fluid oz., powdered ginger, 1½ oz., aromatic spirit of ammonia, 1½ fluid oz. Mix with a rather large quantity of warm gruel. Give slowly and carefully by horn. Follow with ½ pint of linseed oil for the purpose of lubricating the passages, and if there be no relief after 12 hours, repeat the first dose or give 2 pints of castor oil.

INDIGESTION

Is caused by errors in diet. Cattle should be supplied with food which requires remastication, such as hay, grass, or straw, in addition to any more nutritious foods. It seems to be caused by unwholesome herbage or acrid or diseased vegetables, such as decayed turnips. The bowels are irregular, the coat stares, and parts of the cud, while being chewed, are dropped. A pailful of thick, green fluid may be thus lost in two hours. Flesh is lost, the secretion of milk is checked and then stopped, the appetite is impaired, capricious, and finally lost. Poverty of blood and dysentery follow.

Remedy.—Each ox should receive a draft containing 14 oz. Epsom salt, 1½ oz. gentian, and 1½ oz. bicarbonate potassium, mixed, and given in a pint of warm linseed gruel. For about 6 days 6 drams bicarbonate potassium should be mixed morning and evening with the food of each animal; or, if preferred, the powdered salt may be mixed with 1½ oz. of gentian, and given as a draft in gruel or linseed tea. If possible, take cattle to a high, dry, and large pasture, or make an entire change of food at least. Sound roots, good hay, with oil cake, corn, or bran. It is often well to feed little or no green food for a time in the case of animals which have been on grass.

There is a very severe kind of indigestion of calves known as

GASTRO-ENTERITIS.

It is caused by too much milk, and may result in inflammation of the stomach and intestines, causing an acrid discharge called 'white scour.' The bowels may, however, be constipated.

Give alkalies in rather large doses. If diarrhea comes on, stimulant tonics and cordials are useful in addition to more active medicines. Diminish the supply of milk ⅓. and substitute linseed gruel.

Young calves sometimes suffer on account of the presence of hair balls. These may be broken up by the movements of the stomach. If distress is great, relieve with carbonate of ammonium or other stimulant. Trocar rumen if necessary.

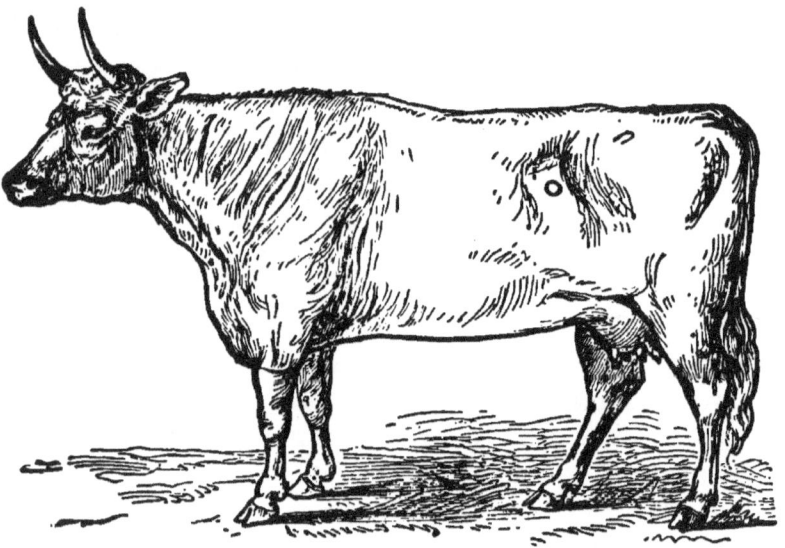

Fig. 109. The spot to trocar the rumen or paunch.

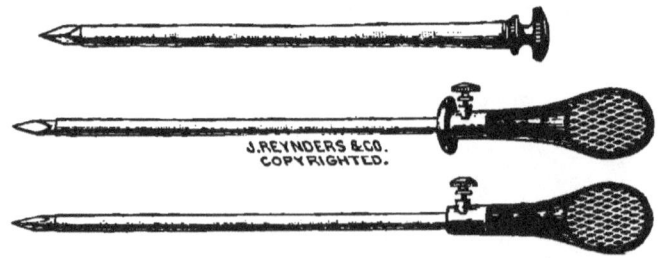

Fig. 110. Trocars.

In calves which have been partially weaned, the abomasum may be overloaded with food, the first and third stomachs not having gained the power of properly preparing the food for it. This may cause constipation. Give oil, be the bowels loose or confined.

Chronic Indigestion may be caused by irregular feeding, bad food, lack of exercise and ventilation, exposure, internal parasites or foreign bodies, &c. As in the horse, the appetite is depraved; the coat stares; the skin feels harsh and dry; the feces are small, hard, dry, and glazed with mucus; the flanks may be now hollow, now swollen; flesh is lost; the animal has a tucked up appearance, &c.; besides which rheumatism, tuberculosis, diarrhea, &c., may supervene.

Remedy.—Change diet, surrounding conditions, &c., as in acute indigestion. Give 14 to 16 oz. Epsom salt, followed by stimulants and tonics. A draft of bicarbonate sodium, 2 oz., sulphur, ½ oz., ginger, ½ oz., gentian, 1 oz., mixed with pint warm water, twice daily, is sometimes beneficial. Puncturing the rumen is sometimes necessary.

SIMPLE COLIC

Is very rare. When severe, all treatment can be avoided, if the animal is in good condition, by slaughtering for the market. The actions of the ox are similar to those of the horse. Many are the same. (See page 103.)

Remedy.—Epsom salt, 16 oz. for full-grown ox. Injections. If plethoric, bleed. Drafts: 1. Aromatic spirit ammonia, 2 fluid oz., tincture opium, 2 fluid oz. Repeat dose in an hour and a half if necessary. 2. Oil turpentine, ½ fluid oz., tincture opium, 1½ fluid oz., spirit nitrous ether, 2 fluid oz., every 4 hours.

FLATULENT (GAS) COLIC

Is also rare. The symptoms are not so severe, but are more continuous than those of simple colic. Sometimes there is distention of the right side of the belly.

Remedy.—Full dose of physic. Walk a little. Rub

right side. Injections and manual exploration of rectum. Draft: Solution ammonia, 1 fluid oz., spirit chloroform, 1 fluid oz., water in proportion, every 4 hours.

CONSTIPATION,

Like colic, is usually merely a symptom of disease. There is usually redness of the lining membrane of the bowels, and also of the eyes and nose. The disorder, as a rule, is due to some impediment, as strictures or engorgements of the stomach or intestines, tumors within the bowels or pressure on them from the outside, volvulus, intussusception, various concretions, &c.

Remedy.—Soft food. Give a laxative now and then. Mild cases often require only injections and bran, linseed, herbage, and roots. In severe cases, give 14 or 16 oz. Epsom salt.

DIARRHEA

Is due to many causes, and like colic and constipation, is often only a symptom of disease. It is a serious affection, and to be treated intelligently and effectively the cause should be ascertained. It may be caused by inflammation, maldigestion, bad food or water, malignant catarrh, epizootic pleuro-pneumonia, cattle plague, an-

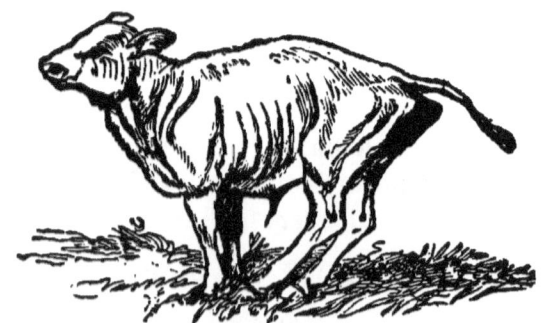

Fig. 111. Diarrhea.

thrax, tuberculosis, &c. There may be severe pain. The appetite is either diminished or depraved. Urine scanty.

If the disease is due to increased activity of the liver, whereby a large quantity of bile is discharged into the small intestine, the feces are dark brown in color, watery, and profuse; if from bad milk or too much milk, they are light colored; if to blood diseases, they are often black and fetid; if to disorder of the pancreas, they are usually light colored.

Remedy.—Powdered opium, 2 drams, catechu, 2 drams, galls, 2 drams, prepared chalk, 1 oz., water, 1 pint, twice daily.

Catechu, 2 drams, camphor, 2 drams, powdered bael fruit, 2 oz., powdered opium, 2 drams, mucilage of starch, 1 pint, twice daily.

For calves: Pepsine, 20 grains, diluted hydrochloric acid, 30 drops, sulphate cinchonine, $7\frac{1}{2}$ grains, water or mucilage of starch, 1 pint, 2 or 3 times daily.

Diluted sulphuric acid, 30 drops, tincture catechu, 2 drams, spirit chloroform, 30 drops, water or mucilage of starch, 1 pint, 3 or 4 times daily.

Salicylate bismuth in 2-dram doses; also salicylate iron.

DYSENTERY,

Inflammation of the lining membrane of the large in-

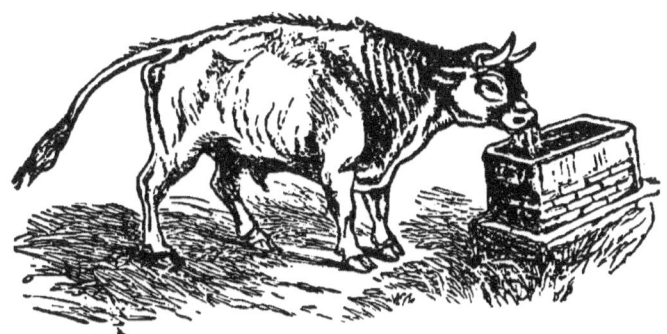

Fig. 112. Acute Dysentery.

testines, often follows diarrhea. It may be accompanied by ulceration. It is either acute or chronic. It is due to bad food, exposure, poison, complication with other diseases, &c.

Symptoms.—Abdominal pain; back arched; constantly straining, passing a small quantity of watery material, tinged with blood; there may be vesicles in the nostrils; coat dry and staring; mucous membranes pallid; ears hung; eyes dull, glassy, sunken; rectum protrudes, &c.

Remedy.—Ipecac, ½ oz., powdered opium, 2 drams, chalk, 2 oz., galls, 2 oz. Mix well and add a pint of warm water or gruel, and give 3 times daily till cured.

INFLAMMATION OF THE INTESTINES (ENTERITIS),

Is rare. It usually occurs among working oxen. It may be caused by too much blood, exposure, drinking cold water when heated, drastic purges, engorgement, &c.

Symptoms.—Pressure on abdomen or loins causes pain; feces often dry and in small quantities; toward the end there may be a little stream of very offensive liquid excrement, which has forced its way through the hard mass of feces by which the rectum is distended; acute febrile symptoms supervene; stands in one place with muzzle protruded; hind limbs become weak; breathing quickened; occasional tremors; excessive thirst; no appetite; moans; grinds teeth; looks at right flank; rectum hot. Other symptoms are like those of colic.

Remedy.—No purging. If plethoric, bleed and repeat if necessary, taking even a gallon. Stimulate belly with rugs wrung out of hot water, renewed at intervals, and by liniments. Give thin, warm gruel with a little linseed oil. Draft: Tincture opium, 2 oz., tincture aconite (V. P.), 40 drops, every 3 or 4 hours. Impacted feces may be removed manually. Anodyne and mucilaginous injections may be very advantageous. Assuage thirst with nitrated water.

V. P. means Veterinary Pharmacopœia (Gresswell's).

INFLAMMATION OF THE PERITONEUM (PERITONITIS),

Is a rare but serious disease. The peritoneum invests the intestines, stomach, liver, spleen, kidneys, &c. The symptoms resemble those of the same disease in the horse, namely: At first stands in a very dejected manner; repeated fits of trembling or shivering, as from cold, followed by a hot stage, throughout which the tremors particularly affect the hind legs and flanks; rumination suspended and appetite lost; ears, horns, and extremities cold; bowels acutely constipated, in some cases giving way to diarrhea, which may be profuse and watery or even bloody; abdomen swollen, tense, and tender near the originally injured or diseased part; urine deficient and highly colored; pulse hard, frequent, wiry; nostrils dilated; respiration labored, quick, catching, but motion confined to chest, abdomen being fixed; looks at flank, crouches, paws, moans, grinds teeth; pulse has become softer, weaker, smaller, while breathing is slower and less painful and labored; membranes pale; eyes sunken; ox stands crouching, with feet close together; coldness of extremities, &c., increases; temperature suddenly declines from 104 or 105° F. to 97 or 95° F.; abdomen falls and is fuller and rounder; less pain and colic; pulse becomes smaller, more rapid, until it cannot be felt. Death occurs in 4 or 5 days from the first appearance of the disease.

Remedy.—No purging or bleeding. Draft: Tincture opium, 2 oz., tincture aconite (V. P.), 40 drops, spirit chloroform, ½ oz., water in proportion, every 6 hours. Injections every 4 hours till bowels are opened. Nutrient injections for weakness.

DROPSY OF THE ABDOMEN (ASCITES),

Is caused by general debility or mechanical impediment to the return of venous blood to the heart, occasioned perhaps by disease of that organ or by disease of the liver, and also by the pressure of a tumor on the portal veins.

The disease is not frequent in the adult, but often occurs in the fetus. The best plan in some cases is to cut, by the aid of the concealed knife, through the abdominal walls of the fetus and let the fluid escape. In the adult the belly is distended, and if one hand be placed against the abdominal wall, while the opposite side is percussed, a wave of fluid may be detected. Dropsical swellings appear on the belly and under the chest. The breathing is thoracic (chest or thorax), and the animal gradually loses blood. The disease is hard to cure.

Remedy.—Nitrate potassium, 2 drams, bicarbonate potassium, 4 drams, oil juniper, 1 dram, spirit nitrous ether, 1 oz., water in proportion. Try to remove the primary cause of the complaint. Tonics. Trocar between the navel and the iliac bone if necessary. Insert instrument gently.

VARIOUS DISORDERS.

Imperforate Anus (absence of anus), occurs mostly in calves. Sometimes the opening is closed with skin. Sometimes the anus itself is perfect, but near the external orifice there is a membranous partition. Sometimes the large intestine may terminate in a 'cul-de-sac' (having one end open only). In the first and second cases, open with crucial incisions. In the third, try to reach the blind end and open it. Then sew the edges of the opened end to the edges of the cutaneous incision.

Distention of the Rectum with hard pellets of meconium (fetal excrements) is sometimes so serious as to necessitate their removal by the oiled finger.

Piles may be removed sometimes by ligature or otherwise. Soft food and an occasional laxative to counteract constipation.

Prolapsus Ani differs from rupture in that the protrusion is through the natural anal opening and consists chiefly of mucous membrane. It results from violent straining, labor pains, or obstruction to the flow of urine. The protruded rectum may become strangulated, take on a bright red hue, and subsequently, owing to effusion, become very much enlarged; then cold and of a purple color.

Remove the cause of the straining, wash the bowel with cold water, and return the part carefully by pressure. If the protruded part is purple, amputate it and stitch the edges. Soft food. Opium if necessary.

Volvulus (twist of an intestine) sometimes follows colic. Open abdomen on the right side and operate on the intestine, if slaughter is not desirable.

Intussusception (entrance of one bowel within another) also follows colic. Rare. Operate as above.

Rupture (hernia) is about the same in the ox as in the horse. In serious cases fatten and slaughter. (For description and treatment, see pages 58, 59.)

DISEASES OF THE LIVER.

THE liver of the ox is situated on the right side, between the third stomach and the diaphragm. Unlike the liver of the horse, it is provided with a gall-bladder large enough to contain several ounces of bile. The bile is liable to become thickened and form calculi as large as a walnut. These are sometimes discharged in the feces, and the pain they cause is thus distinguished from colic.

Anything that interferes with the secretion of bile may cause

JAUNDICE (THE YELLOWS).

Jaundice is easily distinguished by the yellow color of the skin and membranes and the many other signs of disorder which accompany it. But it must not be confounded with the yellowness caused by certain foods. See page 133.

Remedy.—Small quantity of laxative, digestible food. Purge with sulphate of magnesium (Epsom salt), 16 oz., powdered aloes, 8 drams, powdered ginger, $\frac{1}{2}$ oz., mixed with a pint of warm water or gruel.

Draft: Chloride ammonium, 4 drams, bicarbonate potassium, 1 oz., ginger, 4 drams, in pint of warm water, twice daily.

Anything that interferes with the secretion of bile may also cause

INFLAMMATION OF THE LIVER.

A good draft for inflammation of the liver is: Sulphate sodium, 16 oz., caraway seed, 1 oz., in pint warm water, repeated next day if necessary. A 1-dram dose of calomel may be given next day instead of the draft, and half that dose for several days afterward.

Another draft: Tincture aconite (V. P.), 40 drops, chloride ammonium, 6 drams, spirit nitrous ether, 1 fluid oz., water in proportion, 3 times daily till fever abates. Then omit aconite.

Draft for **Torpid Liver:** Diluted nitro-hydrochloric acid, 4 fluid drams, spirit chloroform, ½ fluid oz., tincture euonymin, 1 fluid oz., water in proportion.

DISEASES OF THE CIRCULATORY SYSTEM.

The chief disorders of the circulatory system in cattle are:

Anæmic Palpitation is the result of an attenuated and watery condition of the blood. The murmurs, especially the aortic, produced when the blood is in this state, are softer and more regular than those which arise from disease of the heart. They are often made to cease by a judicious use of tonics. (Gresswell.)

Rupture is rare and fatal. It is caused by overexertion or violence.

Blue Disease (cyanosis) is the result of imperfect closure of the oval foramen (the aperture, in the fetus, between the auricles of the heart), whereby the venous blood from the right side of the heart mingles with the arterial blood of the left side, giving rise to venous pulse and anæmic palpitation, to a blue tinge of the skin and mucous membranes, and to an emaciated and cold state of the body. Moderate exercise may cause death. The young animals usually either die or are killed.

The heart is sometimes found outside the body in calves and lambs. Death usually follows shortly after birth.

Inflammation of the Pericardium (pericarditis) may occur independently or in connection with rheumatism or contagious pleuro-pneumonia. Careful treatment. Death may occur in two days.

Symptoms.—A shivering fit, then becomes dull; pulse accelerated, moderately full and hard, but soon becomes wiry; respiration quickened and labored; nostrils dilated; bowels constipated and urine highly colored; head held low; limbs very cold and usually become dropsical toward the latter stage; sometimes the fluid may be detected inside as well as beneath the chest, extending along the abdomen; pressure on left side causes great pain; flanks hollow; a line runs along the side of the abdomen and chest corresponding to the external oblique muscle, which appears to be unusually contracted, causing the whole abdomen to act irregularly; friction sounds and venous pulse are present, &c. Animals living beyond the sixth day usually recover.

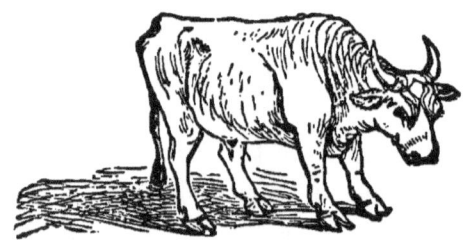

Fig. 113. Inflammation of the Pericardium (Pericarditis).

Remedy.—Drafts: 1. Epsom salt, 12 to 16 oz., calomel, ¼ to 1 dram, croton oil, 5 to 10 drops, ground ginger, 1 to 2 oz. 2. Epsom salt, 12 to 16 oz., croton oil, 10 to 30 drops, ground ginger, 2 oz., molasses, 1 lb., linseed mucilage, 1 quart. 3. Niter, 4 drams, powdered digitalis, 2 drams. Mix and give ¼ part in a pint of gruel every 3 hours.

Inflammation of the Lining Membranes of the Cavities of the Heart (endocarditis) is usually a complication of rheumatism. Careful treatment. Fatten and slaughter.

Inflammation of the Heart (carditis) may be an accompaniment of either pericarditis or endocarditis. The muscular substance of the heart is sometimes inflamed near a deposit or seat of injury. Usually fatal.

Foreign Bodies in the Heart, such as pins, nails, &c., is not uncommon. An animal may live some time with a needle in its heart. If practicable, fatten and slaughter.

Enlargement of the Heart (hypertrophy) is not uncommon.

Embolism is plugging a vessel, such as the iliac arteries, the most usual seat of the disorder, with clots of fibrin (a constituent part of the blood), lymph, &c.

DISEASES OF THE RESPIRATORY SYSTEM.

BLEEDING FROM THE NOSTRILS (EPISTAXIS),

Is the same in cattle as in horses. (See page 76.)

Remedy.—Draft: Tincture perchloride iron, 1½ oz., tincture ergot, 1 oz., water in proportion; or, sulphate iron, 2 drams, powdered ergot, 1 oz., water in proportion.

Cold water and styptic applications or plugging the nostrils may be necessary. If from a polypus, remove with ligature or écraseur.

SIMPLE CATARRH,

The cause and symptoms of which are practically the same in the ox as in the horse, is described on page 70, which see; also 'Malignant Catarrh,' page 231.

Remedy.—Draft: Solution acetate ammonium, 4 oz., bicarbonate potassium, 1 oz., spirit chloroform, ½ oz., water in proportion, 2 or 3 times daily.

Steam with boiling hot water, to which has been added a small proportion of carbolic acid or eucalyptus oil, and put in warm but well ventilated shed.

SORE THROAT (LARYNGITIS),

Like the two preceding disorders, is the same in cattle as in horses. (See page 72.) It differs from catarrh in that the discharge is from the mouth instead of the nostrils.

Remedy.—Tincture belladonna, 6 drams, solution acetate ammonium, 4 oz., water in proportion, 3 times a day. Steam as for catarrh. Gargle: Tincture iodine, 1 part to 20 of water. Liniment for throat: Mustard, 4 oz., oil turpentine, 5 oz.; or, powdered cantharides, 1 oz., olive oil, 8 oz.

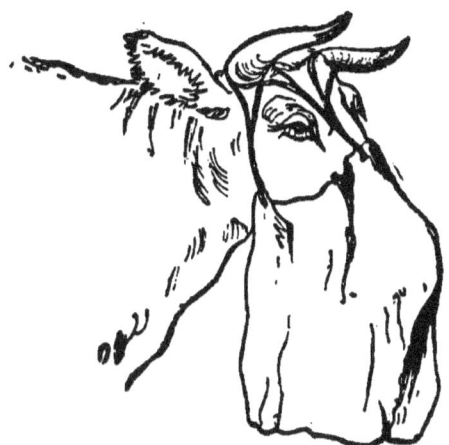

Fig. 114. Steam-bag for Catarrh, Laryngitis, Bronchitis, &c.

INFLAMMATION OF THE BRONCHIAL TUBES AND TRACHEA (BRONCHITIS),

Is of rather frequent occurrence in the ox. It is usually caused by exposure or such mechanical causes as the entry of solid or fluid particles into the air passages, or the presence of parasites in the lungs.

Symptoms.—Pulse hard; respirations greatly increased in number; cough frequent and distressing; mucous membranes purple, owing to want of oxidation; much debility; profuse discharge from nostrils, at first watery, afterward becomes thick; death may result from suffocation.

Remedy.—Maintain strength; careful nursing; pure air. Steam as for catarrh; stimulating applications to chest and throat. Purge if necessary; injections may be given. At a later time it is advisable to give diffusible stimulants, together with vegetable tonics, and allow a liberal diet.

CHRONIC BRONCHITIS

Is frequent. There is a persistent hacking cough, general weakness, a tendency to slight febrile attacks, emaciation, and inability to undergo exertion. The disorder may be associated with asthma, lung inflation, and consolidation of parts of the lung. Although in many cases tonics, quiet, and digestible food will do a great deal of good, slaughter is the best course. The following draft may be given:

Carbonate ammonium, 3 drams, liquor strychninæ hydrochloratis, 2 drams, spirit chloroform, ½ oz., water in proportion, twice daily.

PARASITIC BRONCHITIS,

Also called hoose or husk, frequently occurs in calves under a year old, causing considerable mortality. It is caused by a worm known as the 'Strongylus micrurus,' which is found also in the alimentary canal and in the heart and blood vessels. It is peculiar to wet seasons and low, badly drained lands. Calves kept out late in the autumn, on fields on which animals suffering with the disease have grazed, are especially liable to it. The cough is very forcible and has a special hacking character. It causes the expulsion of stringy mucus, in which parasites or their ova may be seen with a low power of the microscope, and sometimes with the unaided eye. The calves become emaciated and there may be diarrhea. The worms are present in the bronchial tubes and air passages, impeding respiration.

Remedy.—Place the severely affected in comfortable quarters. The bedding on which the discharges fall should be frequently removed and destroyed. Place the slightly affected on high and dry pastures. Pure water and rock salt. Fumigation with the gas from burning sulphur and iodine is strongly recommended, but it should be used cautiously, as the parasites can stand more perhaps than the calves.

PNEUMONIA (Inflammation of the Lungs),

Is not common in cattle as a distinct disease, being usually associated with pleurisy. Pneumonia must not be confounded with the deadly, infectious, and incurable pleuro-pneumonia already described. Simple, non-infectious pneumonia is usually caused by cold, damp or chill. It often takes a favorable turn in 10 days, but death may result in 5, 10, or 14 days.

Symptoms.—Onset usually sudden and characterized by shivering fits; respirations increase from 16 (about the average normal number) to 40 or 70; pulse 70 to 100 (the normal pulse being 40 to 50); temperature is raised several degrees (the normal or natural number being from 101.5 to 102.°5); febrile symptoms very marked; skin dry, parched, hot; thirst marked; as a rule—unlike the horse—sinks to the ground; milk stopped; breathing harsh and loud—distinguished by applying ear to side of chest; cough, though sometimes not marked; bowels constipated; urine scanty and high colored; anxious look; head and neck protruded; as disease progresses, cough, not often frequent, becomes weak, and blood-stained expectoration may be thrown up, &c.

Remedy.—Place in well ventilated box or shed. Purge with a fair dose of Epsom salt in a pint of warm water, and drench with solutions of carbonate and also acetate of ammonium and camphor. Digitalis is also sometimes useful. Apply cloths wrung out of hot water to the chest every hour while acute symptoms last. Then blister on one side with mustard and on the other, if it be also affected, with ointment of cantharides or a strong ammonia or turpentine liniment. It is customary to bleed in acute cases, though aconite, in 45-drop doses, is a **good substitute** for bleeding. In cases that are slaughtered for food, aconite, for obvious reasons, must not be given.

PLEURISY.

Or inflammation of the lining membrane of the chest and lungs, seldom occurs alone in the ox, for it is nearly always accompanied by pneumonia. Like pneumonia, it is usually caused by cold and damp, but it may result from injury or acute rheumatism.

Symptoms.—Fever; pulse 60 to 70, small and firm; breathing: inspiration shallow and short, expiration easier and more prolonged, the chest being fixed as it were, the walls of the belly moving more, thus compensating for the shallow motions of the chest walls; sides of chest and rib spaces tender; by placing ear at side the usual respiratory murmur may be heard, and in addition a loud sound, as of leather creaking and rubbing; dejection and anxiety; eyes half closed; head droops; ears lop; short, painful, hacking cough; appetite diminished or lost, &c.

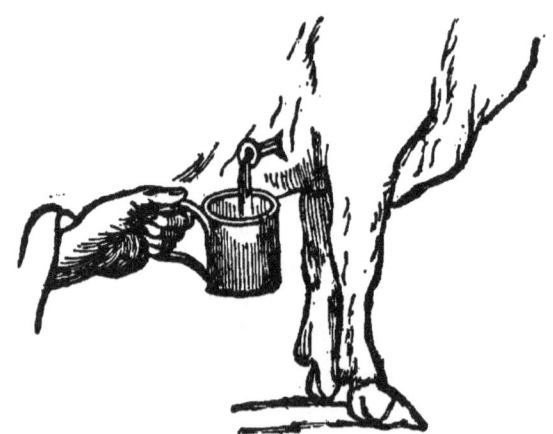

Fig. 115. Tapping the chest for the dropsical stage of Pleurisy.

In many cases the inflammation gradually subsides and the animal slowly recovers; but in others water accumulates in the chest and ends sooner or later in dropsy.

The symptoms change and gradually grow worse. If not relieved by tapping, death soon follows.

Remedy.—No bleeding. After a laxative give a drench of acetate ammonium, camphor, and nitric ether every 4 hours, with the addition of aconite in acute cases in vigorous subjects. Hot cloths and blisters as above for pneumonia. Stimulate with carbonate ammonium, iodide potassium, and digitalis, combined, in dram doses. Tincture perchloride of iron with nux vomica as tonic. Generous diet.

Acute Pulmonary Congestion occasionally results from overwork. It is manifested by extreme difficulty in breathing, profuse cold sweats, cold extremities, very rapid and almost imperceptible pulse, rapid respirations and sometimes a mucous discharge, mingled with a little blood, from the nostrils. The ox lies down, coughs frequently and has a wild look.

Bleeding from the Lungs may be due to acute pulmonary congestion, lung laceration, or consumption. The blood may flow profusely, vary in color, be mixed with mucus, and be discharged from both the nose and mouth.

DISEASES OF THE NERVOUS SYSTEM.

STOMACH STAGGERS

Affords a good illustration of the fact that the brain depends for its well-being on the healthy working of the stomach. When the stomach is very full, the ox may become comatose, so much so perhaps as even to exhibit a tendency to fall down, especially if the head be elevated. The respirations are slow and deep, the pulse slow and full, and the pupils of the eyes dilated. In short, the symptoms may simulate those caused by narcotic poisons.

Remedy.—Give at once a full cathartic dose, and also suitable stimulants. The disorder, as compared to the same in the horse, is rather rare and unimportant.

DELIRIUM

Is not to be looked upon as a disease in itself, but as symptomatic of different kinds of brain disorder. It is met with in inflammation of the brain, in certain blood diseases, in acute indigestion, in impaction of the omasum, and as a result of some forms of poisoning, as, for example, lead.

A delirious ox has a peculiarly wild look of the eye, is excitable—perhaps even frantic and furious; struggles violently against restraint; champs and exudes a frothy saliva, &c. The best remedy is a bullet.

INFLAMMATION OF THE BRAIN (PHRENITIS),

Is not common among cattle, but it is dangerous. It is declining in frequency. It is best distinguished from simple delirium perhaps by the fact that there is a manifestation of acute febrile symptoms. Either the membranes of the brain or the cerebral substance itself may be first attacked. In the former case there is always good reason to fear the extension of this process toward the material of the brain.

When the coverings of the brain are inflamed, spasms, pain, and delirium are shown. The ox is violent, champs the teeth, scrapes, stamps, paws, charges at objects which may be near, displays irregular movements and more or less extreme convulsions. Sometimes these symptoms make their appearance at the first onset of the attack, and the loss of nerve power, the dull and stupid look, the more or less marked paralysis, the loss of sensation, resulting from the extension of inflammation to the brain itself, come on later.

The disorder is peculiar to hot countries and hot seasons, especially if there be a sudden change from cold to heat. Working oxen and the plethoric are the most liable to it. A blow on the head, fracture of the skull, tumors, eating distillery refuse, and perhaps ergotized grasses all seem to be causes.

Symptoms.—Besides those already mentioned, the ox appears sleepy or foolish; pulse and respirations tardy; eyes red and wild looking; head and horns hot; temperature increased, &c.

Remedy.—Bleed freely; cold water to head. Purge, even with croton oil. Hydrocyanic acid subcutaneously. In many cases it is better to slaughter.

For doses, see pages 13 to 29.

MEGRIMS, FITS, STAGGERS (EPILEPSY),

Is peculiar to young and debilitated animals, and may result from lack of blood or certain forms of blood disease. Cattle suffer from gastric vertigo (not unlike epilepsy), and they may have epilepsy, it is said, as a result of long sea voyages or rheumatism. The animal bellows, froths at the mouth, and passes feces and urine involuntarily. Usually the fits soon cease; the ox rises and soon appears healthy again. Fatten and slaughter.

APOPLEXY

Is caused by overdistention and bursting of the blood vessels of the brain and the consequent pressure of the flowing blood on its walls, to fracture of the skull, or to the bursting of an abscess. In a general way the disorder arises from too much blood and from overdriving and excitement in hot weather while in this condition.

Symptoms.—These vary in accordance with the seat of the flowing blood. As a rule they are sudden and marked; looks dull; reels and falls suddenly; unconscious; unable to move or feel; blood vessels of head and neck very full; heart and lungs are the only organs which exhibit life; pulse small and thready; breathing slow, loud, and labored; body covered with cold sweat; mouth open and animal breathing through it almost entirely; eyes widely opened and rolling and staring; pupils dilated; convulsive movements may show themselves, but the muscles are usually soft and flaccid, &c.

Remedy.—Bleed and purge. Strong liniment to loins and spine. If relief does not follow, slaughter.

PARALYSIS

May be due to many different causes, namely, exposure in low, damp pastures, pressure of the fetus on the posterior aorta or the iliac arteries which supply the hind limbs with blood, but which may cease after delivery; poisons, lead palsy, for instance; pressure of tumors on or disease of some part of the nervous system, falls, fractures, &c. (See page 51).

Remedy.—If severe, slaughter. If not, let the animal lie comfortably and be frequently turned to avoid sores. Iodide of iron internally and ointment of biniodide of mercury may be useful. Nutritious, laxative food. Draw urine with catheter frequently. Rub and keep affected part warm.

WATER ON THE BRAIN (HYDROCEPHALUS),

Is caused by the accumulation of watery fluid either between or below the membranes which cover the brain. It usually occurs in the fetus, in which case, in order to deliver the fetus, the enormous head is tapped with a

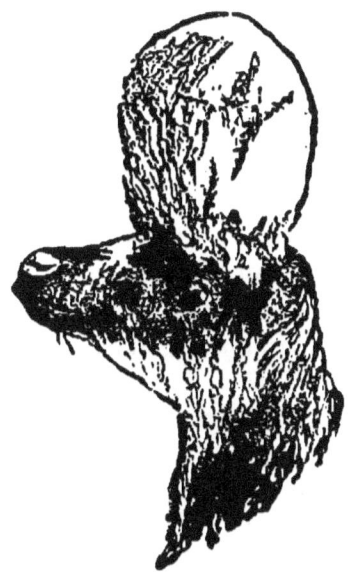

Fig. 116. Hydrocephalus.

trocar (with long canula) or a knife. The head collapses. The disorder may also appear after birth.

The same parasite that afflicts the brain of sheep may afflict cattle. The disorder is known as 'turnsick.' Trephining may be tried.

MILK FEVER OR PARTURIENT APOPLEXY

May occur in three days after calving, though it is said to come on before calving, and even several weeks afterward. It often manifests itself after an easy delivery, in warm weather, in plethoric subjects, in good milkers, and in old animals; seldom before the third calf; usually after the fifth. A cow that once suffers is liable to suffer again.

Symptoms.—Restless; raises first one hind foot then the other, but not disposed to walk; if forced to do so, staggers; appetite lost; no milk; eyes stare; hind limbs give way; falls; eyes now bloodshot, protruded, and insensible to touch; general loss of sensation and voluntary motion; pulse full, soft, slow, but as disease progresses becomes faster, smaller, and finally imperceptible; breathing slow and after a time stertorous; mucous membranes purple; head and horns hot; perhaps delirious; head pitched about, or the animal may lapse into a state of coma; bowels and urinary organs stopped; belly swollen with wind, &c.

Remedy.—Bleed. Purge with Epsom salt, 12 to 16 oz., powdered ginger, $\frac{1}{2}$ oz., in pint warm water. Draft: Carbonate ammonium, 4 drams, powdered ergot, 1 oz., whisky or brandy, 6 oz., in pint warm water, every 4 hours. Inject ergotin hypodermically—15 or 20 grains. Rub spine with liniment of ammonia, 1 part, compound liniment of camphor, 1 part. Don't use liniment of belladonna. Apply wet pack or ice bag to head. Milk regularly. Draw urine with catheter. Digestible, laxative food.

Cows sometimes suffer with a kind of general nervous debility during the latter period of pregnancy. They are unable to rise, the body is cold, the pulse weak, and bowels usually constipated. The disorder may persist after delivery.

Remedy.—Injections for bowels; keep body warm; maintain strength; stimulate and rub back.

Cerebro-Spinal Meningitis, so-called, may follow calving. The cow stands and is free of coma. The bowels may be only slightly deranged, or there may be a fetid diarrhea. The patient may die of apoplexy in 4 or 5 days, or may gradually recover.

Softening of the Spinal Cord (myelitis) is not frequent in the ox. It usually accompanies tetanus (commonly called lock-jaw).

Stringhalt sometimes occurs. In one case, where a number of animals were affected, it was attributed to burnt ale.

DISEASES OF THE URINARY SYSTEM.

DIABETES

Is rare in the ox. It is practically the same in the ox as in the horse. (See page 63.)

Remedy.—Change food; nutritious diet with a fair quantity of water. Gentle laxative. Tincture of iodine. Iodide potassium in drinking water. Vegetable tonics.

For doses, see pages 13 to 29.

ALBUMINOUS URINE (ALBUMINURIA),

Means the presence of albumen in the urine, the microscope revealing "spherical, epithelial cells and granular matter." It is usually the result of cold, injuries, errors of diet, such as too poor or too rich food and congestion or inflammation of some part of the urinary tract.

Remedy.—House well; good, digestible food. Mustard to loins sometimes beneficial. Cupping over loins in acute inflammation of kidneys. Purges and injections if necessary. Digitalis, if ordered by surgeon.

RED WATER, BLACK WATER, BLOODY URINE, MUIR ILL, &c.,

Are different names for a disease characterized by the emission of red-chocolate or black urine, containing albumen and the coloring matter of the blood in a broken or disintegrated condition.

The disease is divided into two kinds—parturient and non-parturient. The former occurs eight or ten days after calving. It is believed to be caused by "a special coccus" (mite), having "a diameter of about half a millimeter," but it is also attributed to impoverished pastures, heathy moors, overfeeding on turnips, &c.

Symptoms.—Great prostration; febrile excitement; palpitation of heart; double, trembling pulse; pallor of mucous membranes; diarrhea followed by obstinate constipation.

Remedy.—Change diet; restrict supply of roots. Saline purge; stomachics and bitters. Iron salts, turpentine, ammonia chloride. For doses, see pages 13 to 29.

INFLAMMATION OF THE KIDNEYS (NEPHRITIS),

Is rare and seems to be confined to working oxen. It may be caused by irritating diuretics, injuries, calculus concretions, &c. (See page 115).

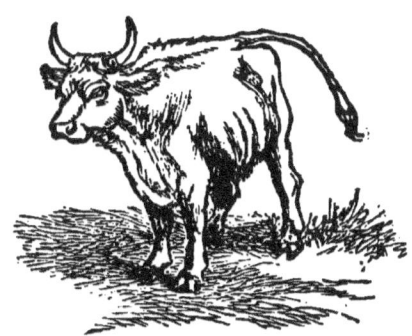

Fig. 117. Nephritis.

Remedy.—Tincture aconite (V. P.), 40 drops, solution acetate ammonium, 4 oz., water in proportion, 3 times a day. Warm injections and purges at outset. Sheep skin or other covering over loins. Bleed if necessary.

Congestion of the Kidneys results from interference with the heart's action or the pulmonary circulation, from which fact it derives its importance.

Uræmia is the more or less complete cessation of the excretion of the waste products of the body which the kidneys ought to separate from the blood. (Gresswell.)

It is a serious disease, as the function ordinarily performed by the kidneys devolves on the skin, bowels, and liver. The blood contains an excess of waste products. The disease follows inflammation of the kidneys.

SUPPRESSION OF URINE

May be complete, though rarely, owing to acute inflammation of the kidneys. It is often partly suppressed in acute febrile diseases. In certain febrile states there may be a deficient secretion of urine, and what is passed will probably be of high specific gravity. The disorder occurs in draft oxen, in dry countries, and in cattle kept on dry pastures in hot, dry weather. Working oxen, fed on dry food, should have about seven gallons of water daily. Those at pasture should be well supplied also.

RETENTION OF URINE

May arise from obstruction or lack of expulsive power, as in paralysis. As a rule the ox is very irritable; lashes tail; lifts hind limbs; lies down often perhaps; tries to pass water; looks at flanks. Sometimes, however, the bladder may burst without manifestation of much pain. Pass catheter and treat according to circumstances.

The name **dysuria** is given to the painful expulsion of urine, and **strangury** to its passage drop by drop, as in spasm or inflammation of the neck of the bladder.

A previous condition of the urachus (canal) may cause constant dribbling of urine through the navel. Ligature or stitch. It is most frequent in prematurely born calves.

INFLAMMATION OF THE BLADDER (CYSTITIS),

Is rare. It may arise from the use of cantharides or injuries. The whole bladder or its neck only may be implicated. There is retention of urine, which, when drawn off with a catheter, is found to contain albumen.

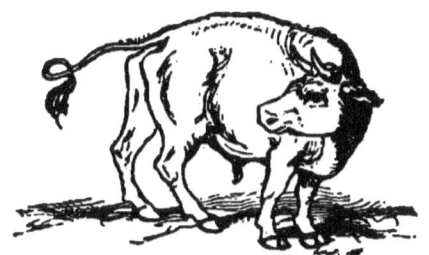

Fig. 118. Cystitis.

Remedy.—Give plenty of watery gruel and nothing else, and apply warm or cold water to the abdomen. Inject an infusion of poppies into the bladder if it can be done without increasing the inflammation.

Stones or Calculus Concretions occur in the kidneys, bladder, urethra, &c., of the ox much the same as in the horse, and are treated, when treated at all, in a similar way. In serious cases slaughter is preferable to treatment. (See page 118.)

Inversion of the Bladder (in the cow) may be caused by excessive labor pains. The organ may be returned after the pains have ceased, but it is usually better to slaughter.

Parasites have been found in the kidneys of the ox.

DISEASES OF THE SKIN.

ERYTHEMA

Consists in a bright redness, diffused generally over the skin, and more or less regularly exhibited. When pressure is applied, this redness disappears, but is soon renewed after the pressure is withdrawn. The disease is rarely seen for many days as a simple erythema, except in parts infected by parasites, for it becomes complicated by the formation of vesicles or even pustules, the discharge from which will mat the hair. The skin may ulcerate and slough off in parts. In some cases the disease remains simple, the cuticle is shed, and health returns. In fatal cases of simple erythema, the redness is confined to the outer layer of the skin, the deeper part as a rule not being much affected.

Simple erythema may become chronic, especially on the teats of cows and sheep. The skin cracks and exudes a thin, gelatinous fluid, which may infect the lips of the calf or lamb.

Remedy.—Begin the treatment of chronic erythema with a laxative; then give liquor arsenicalis, 3 drams, bicarbonate potassium, 1 oz., water, 1 pint, twice a day, after food.

Erythema of the Udder seems to be caused by a constitutional specific infection, the vesicles formed containing matter which causes scarlet fever in man. When severe, handling the teats causes great pain. The milk should be drawn with a siphon and rejected. Remove the calf and dress its mouth if affected.

Remedy.—Ointment: Extract belladonna, 1 part, boric acid, 2 parts, carbolic acid, ½ part, benzolated lard, 13 parts. Ointment of eucalyptus or salicylic acid is also good. Support udder with bandage if necessary.

Compare the above and all other skin diseases of cattle with those of the horse, pages 157 to 176.

ECZEMA

Consists in vesicles in certain parts of the skin, causing denudation of the hair. There is much itching and rubbing, the latter rendering the parts raw. Luxuriant growths of vesicles succeed each other. If the disease becomes chronic, the skin thickens and cracks, and the fissures may even become long, sluggish ulcers. The

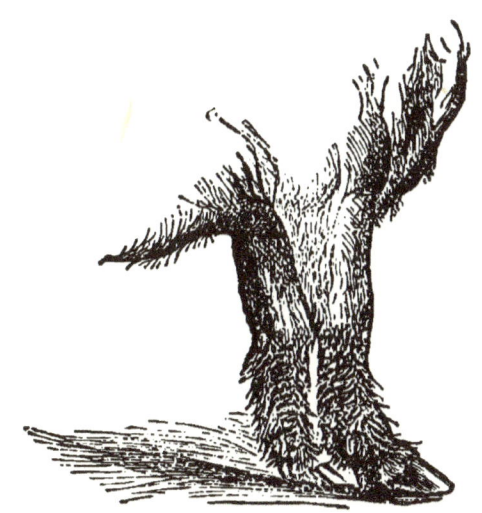

Fig. 119. Rat-tails of chronic Eczema.

growths called rat-tails may be produced, especially on the legs. Even the hoofs may slough, so virulent is the disease.

Remedy.—Comfortable quarters, give a laxative; dress parts with a lead and morphia (morphine) preparation. Good food; cleanliness.

ERYSIPELAS

Affects the whole thickness of the skin, sometimes involving the subcutaneous tissue also. Pain and febrile symptoms are exhibited. It is caused by injuries, strong external applications, burns, scalds, &c. The skin is very red, which does not disappear on pressure. The inflammation may disappear or it may end in ulceration, mortification, or gangrene.

Remedy.—Draft: Tincture perchloride of iron, 1½ oz., spirit chloroform, ½ oz., water in proportion, every 4 hours; or, tincture aconite (V. P.), 40 drops, chlorate potassium, 3 drams, water in proportion, every 6 hours.

HERPES CIRCINATUS

Consists in vesicles similar to those of eczema, which arrange themselves in a gradually widening ring or rings.

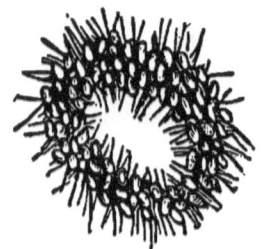
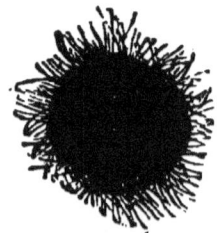

Fig. 120. Vesicles forming.

Fig. 121. Appearance after Vesicles have burst or evaporated.

The vesicles burst, the fluid drying and forming scabs in eight or nine days. The redness of the skin beneath gradually dies away.

For remedy, see page 162.

SORE LIPS (IMPETIGO LABIALIS),

Occur in calves, lambs, goats, and pigs. Sometimes the face and lips of older animals at grass are affected. In calves the upper lip suffers especially, the eruptions ex-

SKIN DISEASES. 277

tending to the membranes of the mouth and nostrils. The disease may possibly be caused by the richness of the milk or by acrid plants.

Change diet. Apply suitable ointment. A purge may be useful.

NETTLE-RASH (URTICARIA),

Consists in numerous eruptions, averaging about two and a half inches in diameter. There is great itching, some increase of temperature, but little or no tenderness or fever. The hair is shed in a few days, leaving bald patches. The eruptions appear suddenly, and usually disappear in about twelve days. Cattle that have been badly kept in the winter and have become rapidly plethoric are most liable to the disease in summer.

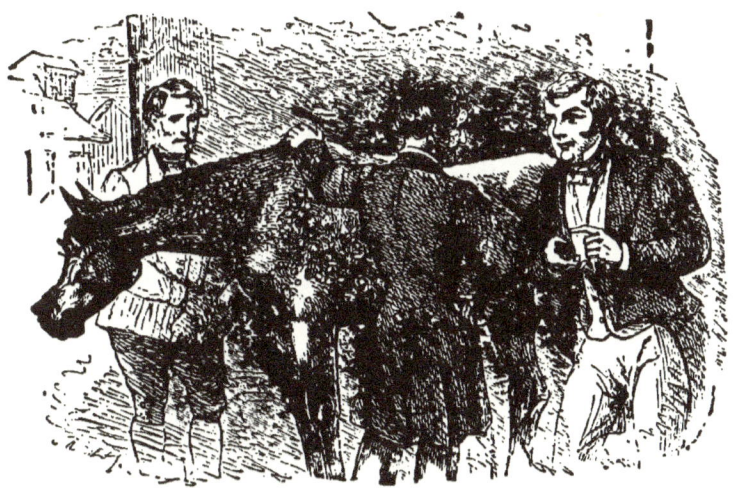

Fig. 122. Nettle-Rash in the horse, the same as in the ox.

Remedy.—Strong saline purge. Paint patches with lotion of glycerine, carbonate of sodium, and laudanum. Sulphur and bicarbonate of potassium in food. Cleanliness, comfort.

Draft: Bicarbonate potassium, $\frac{1}{4}$ oz., bicarbonate sodium, ½ oz., nitrate potassium, ½ oz., water in proportion, twice daily.

PRURIGO

Is sometimes called 'spring-lice.' It is especially common in the spring. Pimples appear on the body and legs, crusts form, which, with the hair, are shed. Coat stares.

Treat as for nettle-rash.

ELEPHANTIASIS

Is said to be "a blood disease, probably originating in an animal poison, and manifesting its existence either by the deposition of a peculiar albuminous substance in the skin, mucous membrane, and other surface tissues of the body, or by affecting chiefly the nervous centers and the nerves. This double mode of manifestation of the disease

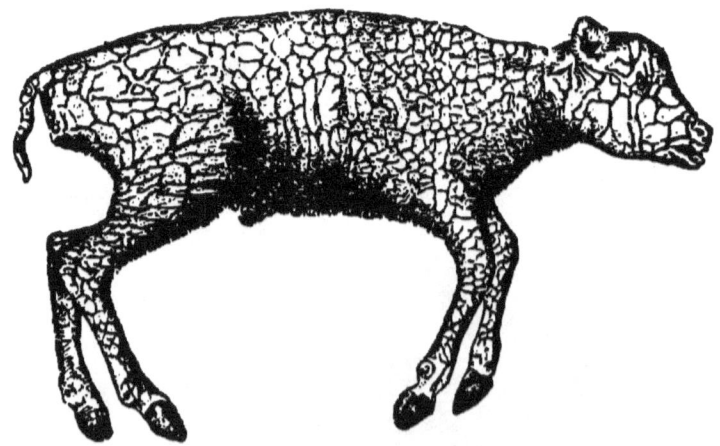

Fig. 123. Elephantiasis.

has caused its division into two kinds—tubercular and anæsthetic." "Both forms are chronic in their course, commencing insidiously, progressing slowly, and lasting for years, sometimes terminating in spontaneous cure and sometimes in death." (Erasmus Wilson.)

For further information and remedies, see page 164.

ECTHYMA,

Which consists of large, prominent, well-defined, and isolated pustules, is rare. The pustules burst, produce a dark-colored scab, which, when shed, leaves a brown stain.

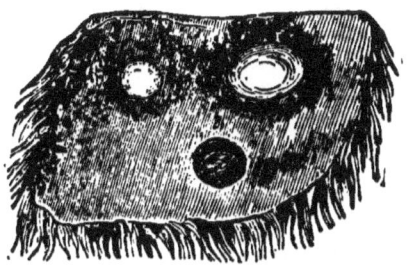

Fig. 124. Ecthyma.

The disease is liable to be mistaken for small-pox. Treat as for nettle-rash.

PEMPHIGUS

Consists in watery bladders, which appear in all parts of the body. In severe cases the bladders may contain pus and blood. They differ in size. Some are as large as a hen's egg. They usually appear and disappear rapidly, sometimes in a few hours. The chronic form, however, may last for months. The bladders burst, or possibly dry up without bursting. Scabs form, which, when shed, reveal a red spot.

Remedy.—Open bladders. Gentle purge; then alkalies. Apply astringent powders, such as starch or the oxide of zinc ointment.

Boils (Furunculus) are caused by intense localized inflammation, involving the subcutaneous areolar tissue and leading to death of a part of the structure, which is expelled as the 'core.' Poultices and fomentations, as in man. Ordinary boils may be left to nature.

Carbuncles differ from boils mainly in the large amount of tissue which dies. Remove dead tissue with knife. Antiseptic dressings. Tonics if necessary. For lists of antiseptics and tonics, see pages 31 and 37 respectively.

Scurf (Pityriasis), is most frequent in young animals. Mild sedative ointment. Change diet.

Nævus means a slight tumor composed of blood vessels. There is usually some enlargement of the superficial layer of the skin.

Warts or Angle Beries may be removed with the knife, ligature, or écraseur. Stop bleeding, if necessary, with hot iron. Some warts are as large as apples.

Baldness (Alopecia), may sometimes be cured by mild but repeated stimulation with tincture of cantharides.

Dropsy (Anasarca), of the subcutaneous tissue of the lower part of the body is not very rare. Careful nursing; hand rubbing; small doses of digitalis.

Emphysema (Inflation), is caused by the escape of gases, resulting from decomposition, into the subcutaneous areolar tissue, as may be seen in some cases of black quarter. Careful feeding. Give stimulant. Rub surface. Make incisions through skin if necessary. Usually there is marked debility.

PARASITIC SKIN DISEASES.

MANGE

Is caused by a minute acarus, peculiar to cattle, which burrows itself in the skin. It usually first appears on the

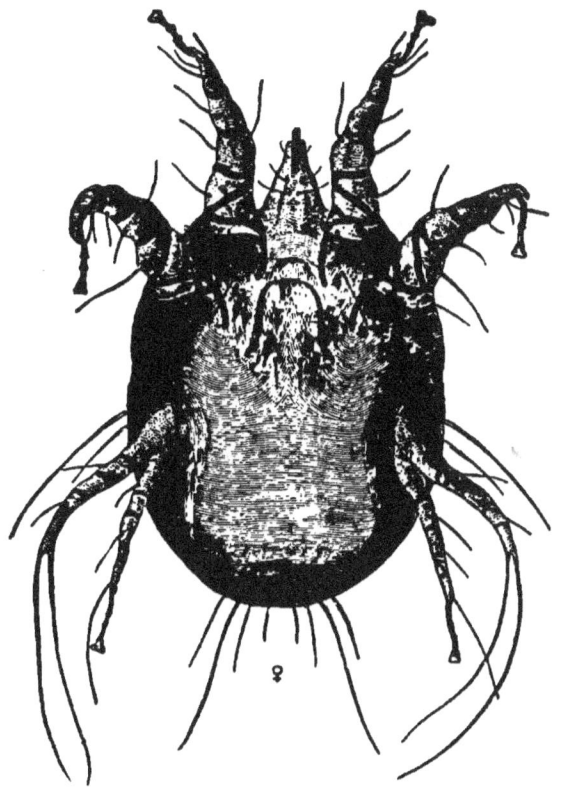

Fig. 125. The mite or acarus known as Dermatodectes bovis. Magnified.

withers and the root of the tail, whence it spreads. The parasite may sometimes be seen in the removed scurf with the naked eye. If it cannot, use the microscope to be sure as to the exact cause of the trouble. The hair of a mangy ox comes off here and there, and the removal of the dry scales reveals small, raw pimples, which discharge a yellowish, watery fluid. In chronic cases the skin becomes thick and folded. The disorder is peculiar to badly kept and debilitated animals.

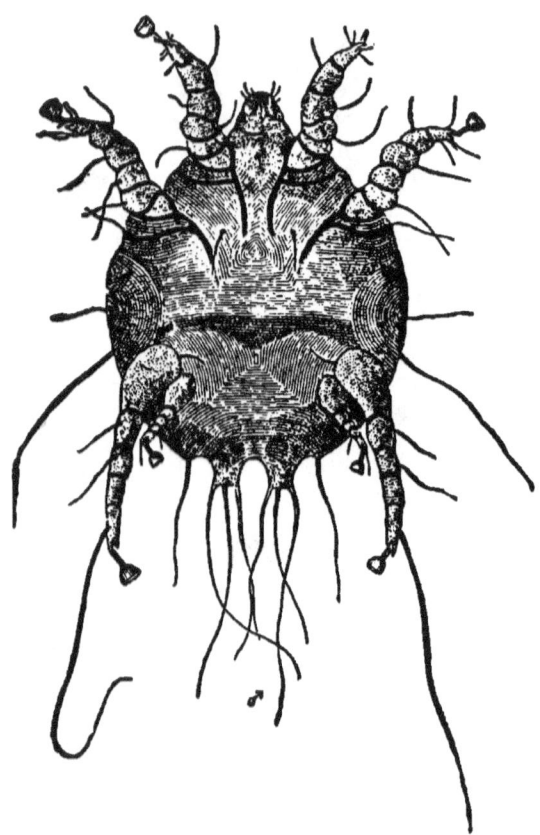

Fig. 126. The mite or acarus known as Symbiotes Bovis. Magnified.

Remedy.—1. Sulphur, 1 oz., lard, 1 oz. 2. Oil of stavesacre, 1 dram, lard, 1 oz. Either of these, or combine the two with 20 grains of white precipitate of mercury. Wash with carbolic acid soap and water before applying ointment. Use ointment every other day till cured. Separate affected animals. Disinfect premises.

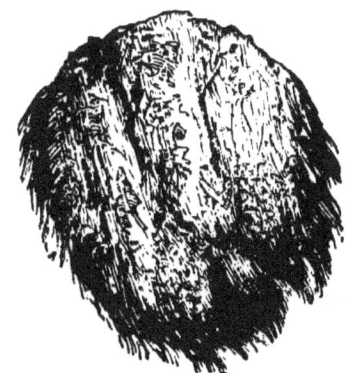

Fig. 127. A piece of mangy skin.

RINGWORM

Is caused by two kinds of fungus. A number of round, scabby patches appear, usually about the head and eyes, giving the animal a hideous look. The rings may unite and form large patches. If the scabs are peeled off, a raw surface is exposed, whence a yellowish fluid exudes, by the drying of which the scabs are formed. The disease is contagious.

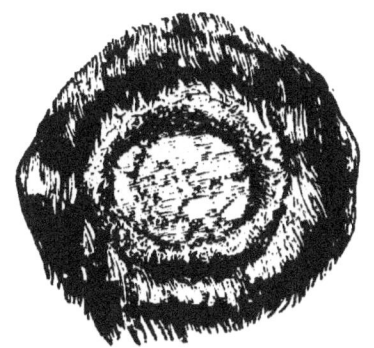 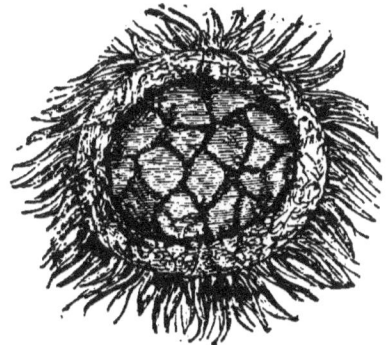

Fig. 128. Ringworm.   Fig. 129. Another specimen same.

Remedy.—Ointment of iodine, or ointment of acid

nitrate of mercury, or oleate of copper, 1 part, lard 5 parts. Lotions: 1. Sulphurous acid, 1 dram, glycerine, 3 drams. 2. Perchloride of mercury, 1 part, water, 500 parts. 3. Vinegar of cantharides.

LICE

May be killed with white precipitate of mercury, 1 part, lard, 12 parts; or, stavesacre seed, $\frac{1}{2}$ oz., soft soap, 2 oz., the bruised seed being boiled with the soap in a pint and a half of water till only one pint remains. Tobacco infusion is also good.

BOT-FLIES, GAD-FLIES, FOUNDER, &C.

THE WARBLE OR BOT-FLY

Is about a half an inch in length and somewhat resembles the bumble-bee. It causes great annoyance. In summer cattle of all ages may be seen galloping furiously about their pastures, tails uplifted, in a state of great excitement. Shortly they stop, look around suspiciously, listen to the buzzing insects, utter a wail, and are off again.

The female lays its eggs on the back of the ox during the latter part of May, and from that time on till the

Fig. 130. Warble or Bot-fly (Œstrus Bovis).

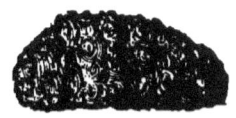

Fig. 131. Pupa (chrysalis state) of same.

first part of August. In December the lumps enlarge, and by spring become about the size of small walnuts. In May the full-grown warble emerges, remaining in chrysalis state till about the middle of June.

Remedy.—The ointment of mercury will destroy the parasite, a portion the size of a pea being enough.

It is desirable that cattle should shelter themselves in sheds. Shallow pools are also serviceable. It is said that the bot-fly will not pursue its victim over water. (Gresswell.)

THE GAD-FLY

Is very different from the warble-fly. It pierces the skin, sucks the blood and causes great pain. (Gresswell.)

Remedy.—Rub with a mixture of 4 oz. of flowers of sulphur, 1 gill spirit of tar, and 1 quart of train oil; or a mixture of spirit of tar, linseed oil, sulphur, and carbolic acid.

FOUL IN THE FOOT

Is usually caused by dampness and is greatly aggravated by dirt and cold. It may, however, be caused by injuries to the hoof or surrounding parts. Fetid discharges often issue from the cleft of the hoof. Parts of the hoof may come off, leaving an exposed, bleeding surface, which may suppurate and even ulcerate. Fungoid granulations may arise and involve the foot and heel. The fetlock may swell and the general health be affected. The horn, if growing irregularly, may split, or it may cause rupture of internal tissues.

Remedy.—Care and cleanliness; place on level floor, with slight backward slope of course. Pare diseased horn and apply linseed poultice. Purge if necessary. Apply any of these ointments:

1. Carbolic acid, 4 drams, lard, 4 oz.
2. Boric acid, 1 part, lard, 7 parts.
3. Sulphate of copper, finely powdered, 1 part, alum, finely powdered, 1 part.
4. Nitrate of copper, 1 part, tar, 6 parts.

Wrap hoof with antiseptic tow or lint. For a list of antiseptics, see page 31.

FOUNDER

Is uncommon, nor is it of much importance in the ox. Purge; rest; cold water applications; salines.

Loss of a hoof may arise from other causes than foul or founder (laminitis), as, for example, catching the foot

DISEASES OF EYES, WOUNDS, FRACTURES, ETC.

in a stage-plank in shipping, unshipping, &c. If time is allowed, a fairly perfect hoof will form.

Cattle are sometimes afflicted with fluke or liver worms. The latter are from 50 to 100 feet long.

Cattle and sheep have practically the same diseases of the eyes as horses, which see (pages 136 to 141). Ordinary cases may be treated to advantage, but in severe cases it is better to fatten and slaughter.

The same may be said of wounds, fractures, sprains, tumors, &c. The bleeding that usually follows broken horns may be stopped by pressure or the actual cautery. Bind a tarred cloth over the orifice.

TEETH, GARGET, ABORTION, ETC.

TEETH.

THE eruption or cutting of the permanent or second set of molar teeth is occasionally a matter of some diffi-

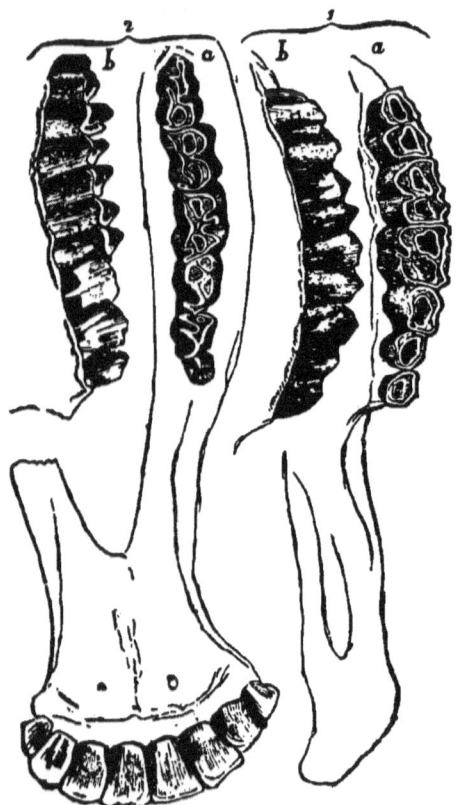

Fig. 132. Teeth of the ox. 1. Upper—*a*, from below; *b*, from side. 2. Lower—*a*, from above; *b*, from side.

culty, owing to the unshed crowns of the temporary or first set of teeth becoming entangled with the new teeth.

This causes irritation and prevents the animal from feeding. In some parts of the country such animals are called "rotten," from their emaciated condition, and perhaps from the fetor emanating from the mouth. When cattle at two years and six months, or about that time, stop

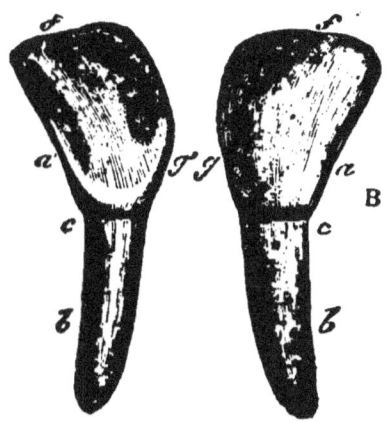

Fig. 133. Incisors of the ox. *a*, crown. *b*, root. *c*, neck. *f*, cutting margin. *g*, inner edge. A, superior surface. B, inferior surface.

feeding, lose condition, or drivel from the mouth, the teeth should be examined, and if the unshed molars are causing irritation, they should be removed with the forceps. Hundreds of young cattle have been sacrificed from this cause—actually dying of starvation. (Williams.)

GARGET (MAMMITIS),

Or inflammation of the udder, may occur shortly or some time after calving. It is often difficult to treat. The whole udder or one or two only of its four quarters may be affected; usually the latter. There is heat, swelling, redness, and pain, and sometimes febrile symptoms. If properly treated, the disease subsides, but severe cases may end in exudation, suppuration, or abscess. A large part of the gland may become indurated and suffer a permanent loss of secreting power. There may be lameness in one hind leg; pulse quick and hard; chewing cud may be suspended, appetite lost, &c.

The disorder may be caused by blows, scratches, or other injuries, and perhaps from plethora at the time of calving. Heifers are especially liable to the disorder, and the heat of summer is said to be an exciting cause.

Remedy.—Bleed and purge if necessary. Foment udder with warm water; apply linseed poultice containing 2 to 4 drams of extract of belladonna. Milk regularly. Draft: Bicarbonate potassium, 1 oz., tincture aconite, 40 drops, water in proportion; or, nitrate potassium, 1 oz., tincture aconite, 40 drops, water in proportion, every 4 hours, and then 3 times daily as long as the temperature remains high.

For chronic hardening inject bicarbonate of potassium, 1 dram, water, 1 oz. Rub with acetic liniment. Draft: Bicarbonate potassium, 1 oz., iodide potassium, 2 drams, water in proportion, twice daily.

Sore and Obstructed Teats are caused by minute tumors and milk stones in the canal of the teat. Pass a silver or other probe. A clean, oiled knitting needle will answer. Warts about the end of the teats should be removed by ligature. Sore or chapped teats are best treated with ointment of turpentine.

ABORTION

Is liable to occur frequently and at almost any period of pregnancy. It is sometimes epizootic. It has many causes, such as all kinds of unsanitary conditions, mechanical injuries, overdriving, innutritious and badly prepared food, ergotized grain and poisonous plants, consumption, sympathy (the sympathy of a well cow with an aborted cow), malformations, blood and other diseases, close in-and-in-breeding, the prolonged use of one bull in a herd, &c. A cow that has once aborted is liable to abort again. Such had better be fattened and killed for food.

Remedy.—Isolate aborted animals; burn, disinfect, or deeply bury fetus and placenta. Disinfect and cleanse premises. Irrigate uterus, vagina, tail, &c., with an effectual germicide, such as corrosive sublimate, 1 part, common salt, 40 parts, clean rain water, 4,000 parts; or, mercuric iodide and potassium iodide, 1 part each, water, 1,000 parts. Use these injections to prevent abortion in cows that have been herded with the aborted. Prevent use of bull with balanitis (inflammation of mucous membrane of penis). Gentle laxative; quiet; tonics.

RETENTION OF THE PLACENTA (THE AFTER-BIRTH),

Often follows abortion, but it also follows an otherwise natural delivery. It may be caused by weakness or contraction of the uterus. Decomposition of the placenta causes blood poisoning and death.

Remedy.—Epsom salt, 16 oz., carbonate ammonium, 4 drams, in 2 pints warm water, repeated next day if necessary. Traction (or attraction) may be applied by the medium of the protruding part of the cord, the efforts made coinciding with the labor pains; or the projecting parts may be rolled round two sticks. If this does not suffice, introduce the hand gently and detach the placental lobes. After removal, wash uterus with chlorinated lime. Gentle laxative if necessary and plenty of good gruel. Brandy, spirit of niter, &c., if necessary.

Inversion of the Bladder is not frequent in cows, but it is usually fatal. The bladder has the appearance of a tumor. The end of the canals which convey the urine from the kidneys to the bladder may be seen on either side; also the escaping urine. In the early stage return is not difficult. If it cannot be returned, slaughter.

Inversion of the Vagina usually occurs in the debilitated and before birth. Bathe with cold water, return part, and use truss till birth-time. Good food.

Inversion of the Uterus is common. Cleanse of dung, straw, &c., and then detach the afterbirth. Place on clean cloth, with a man supporting on each side. Gentle and increasing pressure on neck of uterus· then apply fist to lower part.

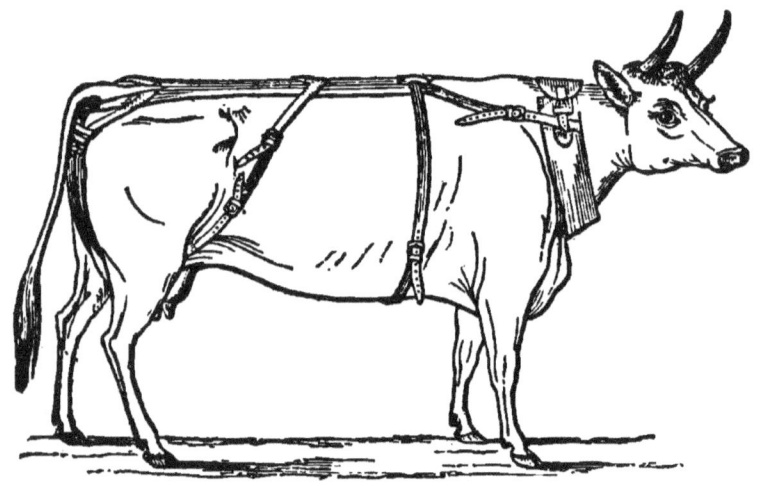

Fig. 134. Truss for Inversion of Uterus (prolapsus uteri).

It may be necessary to cast and place cow on back, the hind parts being somewhat elevated with straw. After return, apply a truss. Give opium if required. In some cases it may be necessary to ligature the neck of the uterus and cut off the remainder. This operation—amputation of the uterus—is of somewhat common occurrence.

Dropsy of the Uterus is not uncommon. The cow looks as if in calf, so distended is the womb with water. The closed mouth of the uterus may be dilated with the finger.

Malformation of the Uterus is seen in hermaphrodite heifers, which are generally sterile.

In a natural birth the fore feet appear first, the head, resting on the fore legs, next. There are many "false presentations," besides which the head of the fetus may be enlarged by water on the brain, or its abdomen may be enlarged by dropsy. Such cases require surgical skill.

Twins are somewhat frequent. When one has been removed, look for another. They usually lie in reverse positions, one being presented in the natural way, the other with its hind legs first. Twins are usually small, and are therefore delivered without much difficulty. They are apt to become fixed together in the genital passages. In such cases, the state of affairs having been ascertained, the fore legs of the naturally presented calf are to be secured with ropes. These being kept tight, the other calf is forced back into the uterus. The first can then be removed in the natural way. The second will usually follow.

Obstructions in the Teats are not rare. In milking the animal, they can be felt as knots along the course of the duct, and the flow will be more or less impeded. These are masses of curdled milk, small tumors attached by pedicles to the mucous membrane, or 'lacteal calculi.' They must be removed, as they tend to produce mammitis (inflammation of the mammary or milk glands). This is not always an easy matter. When not removed, they may be returnable to the contiguous sinuses (cavities), where they will often remain without causing inconvenience.

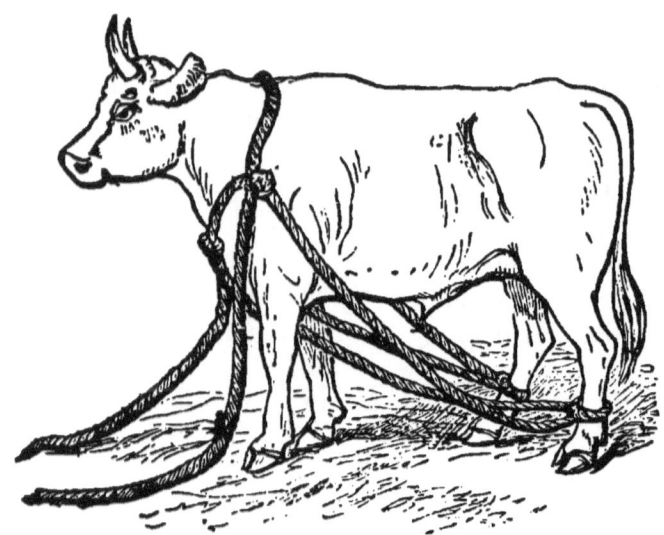

Fig. 135. The ox prepared for casting.

PART III.

THE DISEASES OF SHEEP.

THE diseases of sheep, says Walley, are usually caused by an altered condition of the blood, namely, deficiency in quantity, excess of normal elements, impoverishment and degradation, depraved condition, &c. In-breeding is a predisposing cause of disease. The rams should be changed every year or two. Fatigue, clipping, and exposure to cold wind (sufficient to cause a chill) induce congestion of the lungs. Sheep can stand almost any degree of cold alone, but they cannot stand cold and wet combined. This is especially true of lambs. Cold and moisture arrest the secretion of the *yolk* or greasy matter exuded by the skin, rendering the wool dry and harsh instead of greasy.

Avoid overfeeding and sudden changes of food and management. Also the procreative exhaustion of the rams and the excessive excitement of the ewes. Also filthy, decaying, moldy, or frosted (frozen) food and impure water. Also overforcing the fattening process, especially with such foods as Waterloo cake, cotton cake, turnips, and swedes.

The sheep, like the ox, has four stomachs. The fourth is the true digestive stomach. This complicated digestive apparatus should be aided, when necessary, by health-giving foods, such as oats (crushed preferred), bran, crushed linseed, and ground malt. Corn, beans, peas, and wheat are good when given in their proper place and quantity. Also thousand headed or other cabbage. Mutton grown on ling and heather is sweeter and more satisfying than that of trough or manger-fed sheep. Turnips and swedes alone are very bad, especially when filthy. They produce flesh but no blood.

"I have seen sheep, especially lambing ewes, that have been fed *ad libitum* on swedes, without any complementary food, die in dozens, their carcasses laden with fat, but not a teacupful of blood in the veins of any of them. In the case of breeding ewes, I have seen the recently born lambs the subjects of internal dropsies. Again, I have seen ewes fed in the same way, on swedes which have been forced with artificial manures, especially phosphatic manure, die in dozens from milk fever (so called in some districts), while their lambs have succumbed to joint-ill. Prof. Robertson says he has, by way of experiment, produced these diseases at will." (Walley.)

THRUSH OR APHTHA

Has a benign as well as a malignant form. The benign form usually attacks lambs, and the malignant may be communicated to them by the milk. Both forms are attributed to a fungus, the benign to that known as 'oidium albicans.' The benign is short-lived. It is characterized by a whitish, furred eruption in the mouth, with a little fever and diarrhea.

The malignant form not only has eruptions in the mouth, but also on the lips and about the body, with bleeding ulceration, diarrhea, or dysentery, and even putrefactive fever and abscesses about the head and lungs, constituting pyæmia (purulent contamination of the blood).

Remedy.—Alum, borax, sulphurous acid, chlorine, or

potassium chlorate solutions locally. Electuaries (confections) of oxymel, glycerine, and water, and glyceride of starch. Laxatives, salines, hydrargyrum cum creta for gastric disorder. Tonics. Soft, digestible food.

For doses, see pages 13 to 29.

ERYTHEMA

Is described on pages 157 and 274. If the lambs are allowed to suck, protect the teats with a gutta-percha shield; otherwise they may become very sore. If they do become sore, place the ewes on a scanty pasture apart from the lambs. Rub the teats with boric or salicylic acid ointment night and morning. Cleanse first if necessary.

ECZEMA OF THE LIPS

Is usually attributed to the irritation of fine particles of sand or gravel, aggravated by long-continued wet, but in some instances it may be caused by indigestion or stomach irritation, and probably the irritating action of pollen grain. It is a mild affection, consisting of crops of small bladders on the lips, with some local inflammation and slight fever. If neglected and its cause be unremoved, serious results may follow. The lips become greatly swollen, misshaped, and tender, the skin chapped and ulcerated. Small abscesses form along the side of the face and in the lungs, followed by suppuration of the neck glands. Flesh useless.

Remedy.—Change the pasture, give a little laxative medicine, and smear some protective agent, such as carbolized lard, over the lips.

CARBUNCLE

Is less frequent than eczema, but is common in lambs, especially during the autumn months. It is often called 'hair and hoof' and 'orf.' Like eczema, it is usually of a mild character. If neglected, it may lead to deep-seated inflammation, ultimately causing death by exhaustion or blood poisoning. Its cause is not known, but it may be due to a depraved condition of the blood, as the result of injudicious management, to irritation of the stomach and bowels, to a microscopic parasite acting locally, or to a parasitic product, such as ergot, acting systemically.

The disease first appears as a painful, circumscribed swelling on the coronet or lip, or both. Ulceration of the skin results, and an angry looking sore, associated with considerable thickening of the surrounding tissues, is formed. If properly treated, this sore quickly heals, but if irritated by dirt or otherwise, it takes on unhealthy action, spreads, and becomes very intractable. Treat as for eczema.

ECTHYMA,

Consisting of small, pointed, pustular eruptions, occurs often in the summer time. It causes very little general disturbance, and is of little importance except for the

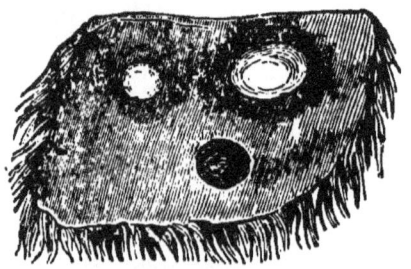

Fig. 136. Ecthyma. Compare with figures 137, 138 (opposite page.)

fact that it may possibly be mistaken for sheep-pox, a very serious disease. The pustules dry up without leaving a scar. The disease is sometimes called acne.

See pages 163, 279 for further information concerning this disease.

SHEEP-POX (VARIOLA OVINÆ),

Is a contagious, infectious, and eruptive disease, analogous to small-pox and cow-pox; said to depend on a

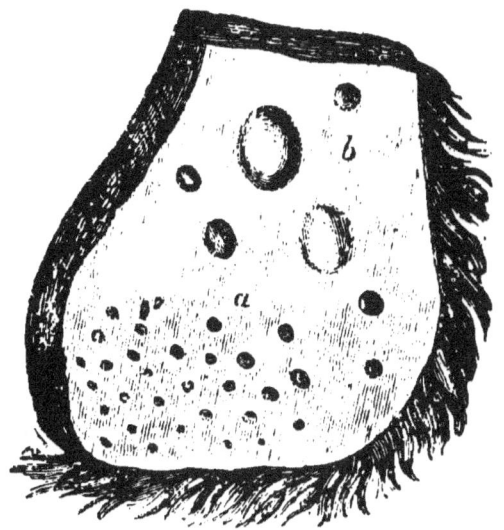

Fig. 137. Sheep-pox. *a*, the eruptive stage. *b*, the pustular stage.

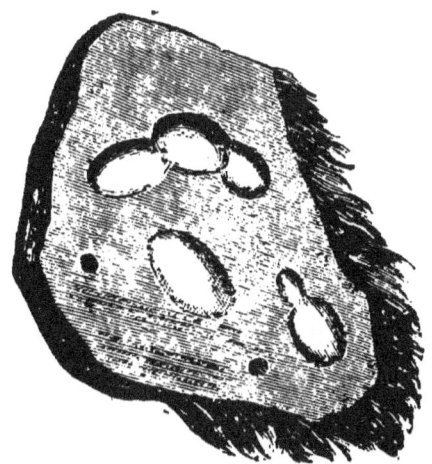

Fig. 138. The Confluent Form (union of two or more pustules).

microbe; runs a definite course, and as a rule occurs but once,

There is both a benign and a malignant form. The malignant form never produces vesicles; the sheep lose their eyes; the wool falls off; the skin cracks in a zigzag manner, and the nostrils become filled with a fetid discharge. In the benign form genuine vesicles appear, which, after the scabs fall, leave pits in the skin, on which the wool never grows again.

According to Prof. Simonds, the disease is not communicable to the cow or to children. Saccho, however, says that 'ovination' is protective against small-pox.

Symptoms.—In 36 to 48 hours temperature rises to 105°, or even 107 or 108°; skin dotted with bright red pimples; eyes bloodshot, and in severe cases the lids are swollen and tears trickle down the face; breathing quick and short; mucous discharge from nostrils, &c.

Remedy.—Isolate healthy and watch them. Good nursing. Gentle aperients; salines. Tonics; stimulants; nutritive, digestible food for convalescents. Inoculation of healthy sheep produces a rather severe and contagious form of the disease.

MALIGNANT CATARRH

Is often very destructive to hill sheep, especially in bad seasons. It is very intractable. Beginning apparently as a simple cold, it is soon followed by destructive inflammation and ulceration of the lining of the nostrils; these in turn by abscesses in the glands of the face and throat; also in the lungs, and, if the animal lives long enough, by wasting and diarrhea. The disease is probably caused by a micrococcus. (Walley.)

Sheep sometimes suffer from simple catarrh, laryngitis, and bronchitis. (See pages 70, 82, 258 &c.) Verminous bronchitis is caused by worms in the air tubes. (See husk.)

MANGE, SCABIES, OR SCAB

Is caused by a parasite (Psoroptes ovis). The parasites cause great irritation and itching. Sheep will rub themselves against anything. To make sure as to the para-

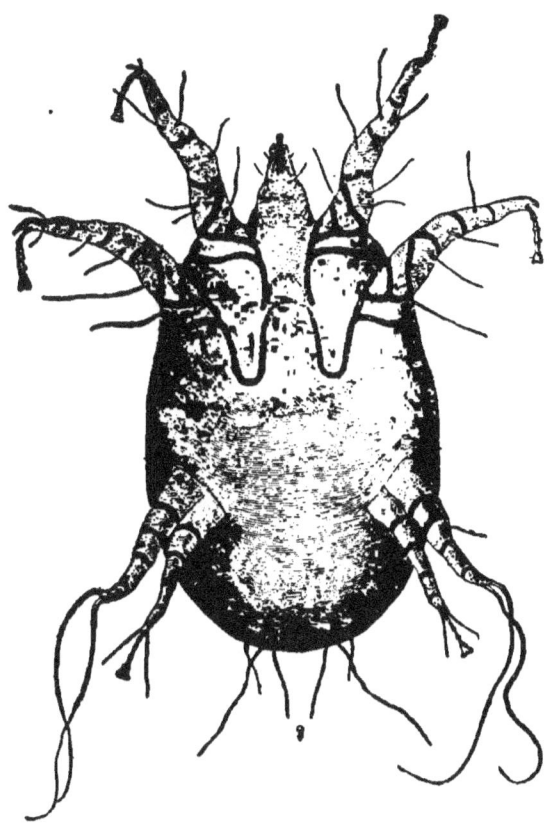

Fig. 139. The mite or acarus known as Dermatodectes ovis. Magnified.

sites, remove a little scurf and examine with a pocket lens or microscope. If neglected the parasites will spread to a whole flock and cause great loss.

Remedy.—Dress with corrosive sublimate, 1 part, common salt, 8 parts, water, 500 parts. Decoction of tobacco, 1 part, water, 40 parts. Stavesacre decoction—1 part to 40 of water—with half of which shake up when using 1 part each of wood tar oil and potassium carbonate. Any of the foregoing, or sulphur, 1 oz., lard, 1 oz.

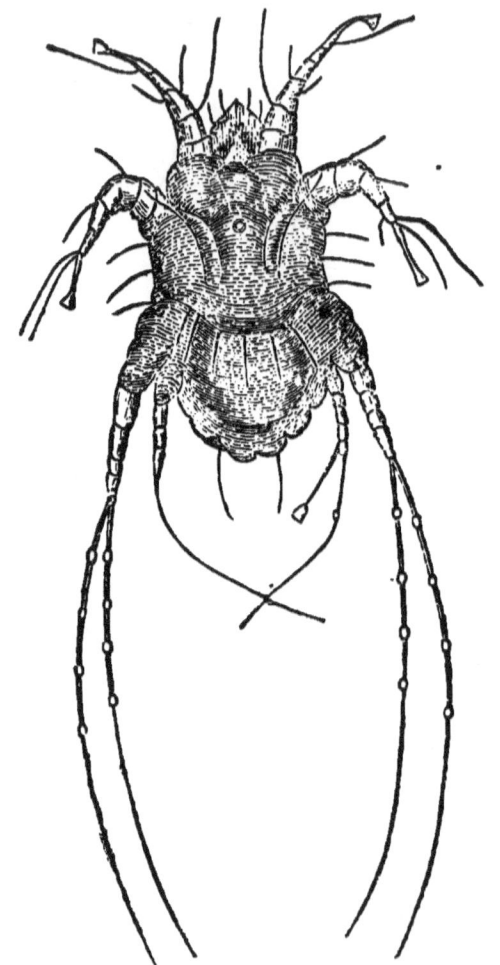

Fig. 140. The mite or acarus known as Sarcoptes ovis, from beneath. Magnified. Compare with Fig. 141, opposite page.

In all bad cases the sheep should be bare shorn and the affected parts well soaked with potash lye before the insecticide is applied. Isolate affected sheep and wash racks, rubbing posts, &c., with corrosive sublimate solution.

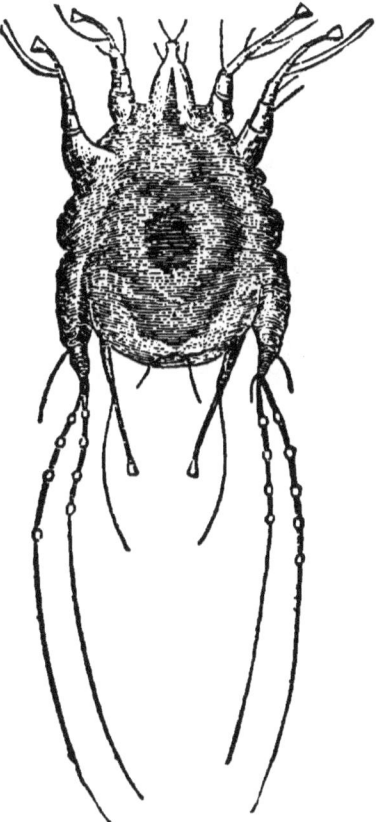

Fig. 141. Same from above.

FOOT-ROT

Is inflammation and ulceration affecting various structures of the foot, and is frequently contagious. (1) Abrasion of horn; inflammation of secreting surfaces of sole or walls, beginning below and extending upward. (2) Inflammation of interdigital structures, with burrowing of discharges under the horn of inner walls of digits, beginning above and extending downward. The latter is the more contagious form.

304   THE DISEASES OF SHEEP.

Williams says the disease is not contagious.

Remedy.—Remove diseased horn and any irritating foreign bodies. Dress with mercuric nitrate solution, zinc

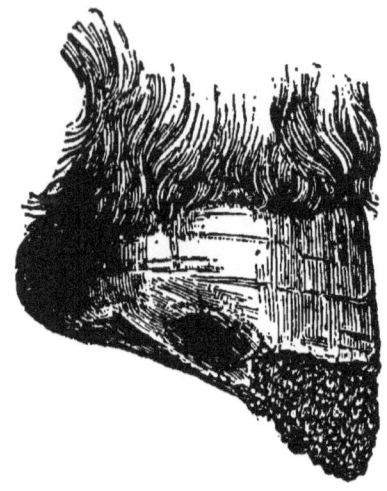

Fig. 142. Confirmed stage of the first form of Foot-Rot.

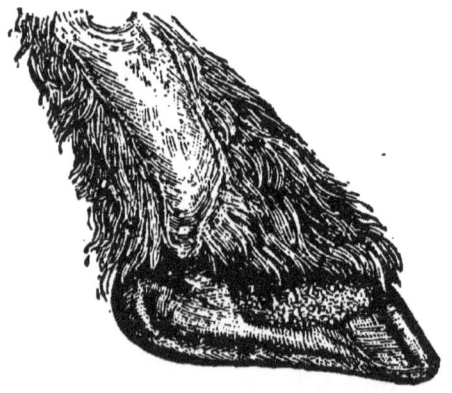

Fig. 143. The condition of the internal wall of the digit in an early stage of the disease.

chloride, carbolic acid, tar oils, or silver nitrate, the strength of the dressings being regulated according to circumstances. Gutta-percha varnish may be sometimes usefully applied over dressing. Walk sheep through wooden trough containing 1 lb. each of arsenic and sodium carbonate and 50 gallons of water; or, 1 part copper sulphate to 50 parts of water. Avoid beans and other forcing food. Transfer flock to dry, upland pastures.

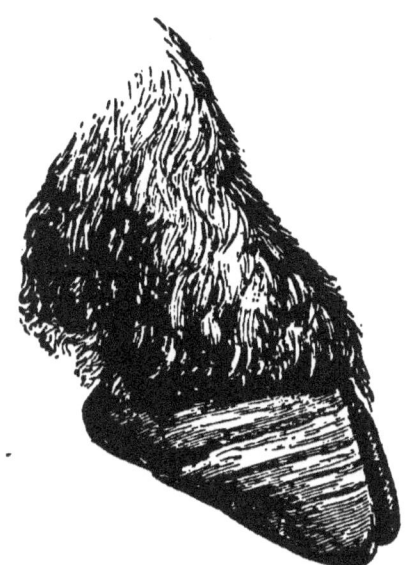
Fig. 144. Foot four weeks after first or febrile stage.

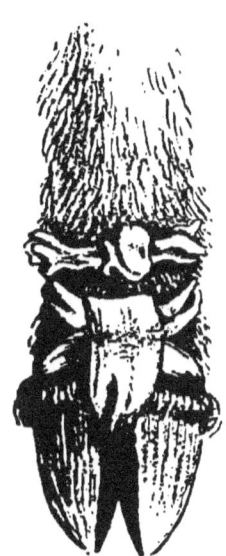
Fig. 145. Bandage for Foot-Rot.

ROT OR FLUKE DISEASE

Is caused by a flat worm known as the fluke (Distoma hepaticum or Fasciola hepaticum), which inhabits the bile ducts of the liver, causing extensive inflammation, from which result various organic changes, such as hardening and softening, leading in the end to destruction of its function and, as a result, wasting, lack of blood, dropsy, diarrhea, and death from exhaustion. When cold nights follow warm days, many die from congestion of the lungs as the result of chill.

The worm is seldom more than an inch in length. It is bisexual (hermaphrodite), and is propagated by eggs, which are passed out with the bile and the dung in countless numbers, often lodging on the grass. If they fall on dry soil, they are harmless; if on wet soil, the disease is propagated to other sheep. The egg is oval in shape, has a lid at one extremity, and contains an embryo which, when matured, is provided with delicate, hair-like processes known as cilia. The lid is lifted, allowing the embryo to escape. The latter at once begins to search for a particular snail (the Limnus truncatulus), whose body it penetrates by the aid of a boring apparatus. It undergoes a series of wonderful changes in form, passing through several generations, until a tadpole-like creature is produced. Emerging, it encysts itself in the lower part of the blades of grass, from whence sheep pick it up in grazing.

Sheep are more susceptible to rot than other animals simply because they bite closer. A hog-mouthed sheep escapes; but many cattle and sometimes, in wet seasons, colts also suffer.

Rot is never seen on dry lands, nor on salt marshes; and even rotting grounds are safe after a frost.

Prevention.—Drain, and thereby kill the snails; salt the pastures, and thereby kill both the snails and embryo worms; slaughter sheep, mixing their excrements with lime or salt; destroy the liver, intestines, &c., totally. Isolate sound sheep.

The disease can be detected early by the sheep thriving very rapidly and by the yellow tinge of the membrane of the eye.

Remedy.—Concentrated, dry food. Common salt and ferrous sulphate dissolved in water, given daily, mixed with bran or crushed grain. Slaughter all marketable sheep.

For doses of 'furrous sulphate' (sulphate of iron), see page 21.

DIARRHEA

In the lamb is caused by unwholesome milk, cold, grass (the sudden change from milk to grass), &c. In severe cases death sometimes results in 24 hours. Full-grown sheep also suffer, especially when the new grass comes on in the spring.

Remedy.—Prepared chalk, 1 oz., powdered catechu, $\frac{1}{2}$ oz., powdered ginger, 2 drams, powdered opium, $\frac{1}{2}$ dram, peppermint water, $\frac{1}{2}$ pint; 1 to 2 tablespoonfuls morning and night. A teaspoonful of laudanum and a tablespoonful of rum or gin, well mixed, is good; repeated in half doses if needed. Also $1\frac{1}{2}$ dram alum in half pint warm water.

DYSENTERY

Usually appears in hot weather, with excess of moisture, on rank pastures, and on overstocked and consequently befouled pastures; in dry summers on lands having stagnant pools of water, with rank growth of grass around their borders.

The exact nature of the disease has not been determined yet even in man, but it is believed to be caused by a fungus. Shepherds entertain such positive views as to its contagiousness as to lead them to smear tar on the nose. They had better smear it on the skin under the tail, or remove the sheep from the contaminated pastures and apply a top dressing of lime or salt.

Remedy.—If there is any prospect of cure, give an ounce of castor oil with about 30 drops of laudanum in a little gruel; repeat if necessary, or give an astringent as for diarrhea. Cleanse with warm water and carbolic acid soap. Dress any sores with carbolic or salicylic acid, or lard mixed with a few drops of spirit of tar. Tempt appetite with well compounded gruel.

CARBUNCULAR FEVER (ANTHRAX),

Is caused, says Walley, by a minute, staff-like organism, termed, from its shape, a bacillus, and belonging to the class of fission (generative) fungi. It is, on the whole, the largest of this class of fungi found in animals, and in the blood streams and tissues multiplies only by fission; but when cultivated in proper media, or, what is of more importance to farmers, when it gains access to suitable soils, it multiplies rapidly by spores, which by various agencies find their way on to vegetables grown on such soils and into drinking water, and produce the disease in other animals that may partake of the contaminated food and water.

These organisms, and particularly their spores, possess a wonderful vitality, and retain their destructive properties for a very considerable period in the earth. Hence the necessity of utterly destroying every part of the carcass, the blood, and internal organs of animals which have died of the disease.

The disease is communicable to man, and is known under various designations in many parts of the world. There is reason to believe that it may be disseminated by artificial manures, and sometimes even by artificial food, as it often appears in situations where it has never been seen before.

Anthrax, which, owing to the dark color of the local lesions, is compared to a burning coal, is the most deadly disease of its class. So-called 'red braxy' is often nothing more or less than anthrax.

'Black-leg' is a disease somewhat allied to anthrax, but the organism that produces it is of a rather different character, and it is much less virulent.

Remedy.—Free scarification of limited external swellings and introduction of antiseptics seem to arrest some slight cases. Intra-venous injection of virus usually insures immunity from attack. Setons produce a condition of the body less favorable to development of micro-organisms. Careful dietary. Removal from exposed, undrained, infected grazings.

Compare above article with pages 225, 226.

STURDY, GID, TURNSICK,

Also known as turnside, goggles, vertigo, &c., is due to a bladder worm in the brain. It is called sturdy because the animal is stupid. A synonymous term in Norfolk, England, is 'dunt.' If the sheep turns to one side or round and round, it is known as turnsick, gid, &c., while, owing to peculiarities of gait, sheep are said to be sailors, trotters, or swervers. The disease is peculiar to cattle also.

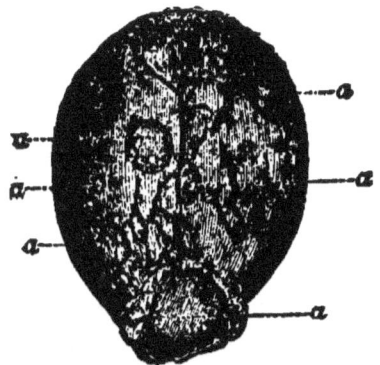 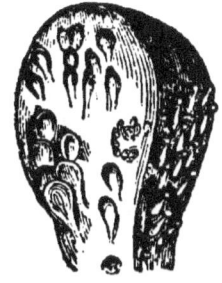

Fig. 146. Brain of sheep, showing hydatids or tapeworm cysts.

Fig. 147. Cyst, showing embryo worms in various stages development.

The bladder worm or hydatid is the immature form of one of the tapeworms of the dog; possibly also the fox. It is known as the many-headed hydatid. Sheep become the victims of it by swallowing the eggs of the tapeworm while grazing. The embryo finds its way to the brain either by the circulation or by boring, and sometimes it gains access to the spinal cord, in the neck, and causes the condition known as thorter-ill.

Prevention consists in destroying the brain instead of throwing it to the dogs. Keep dogs as free from tapeworms as possible.

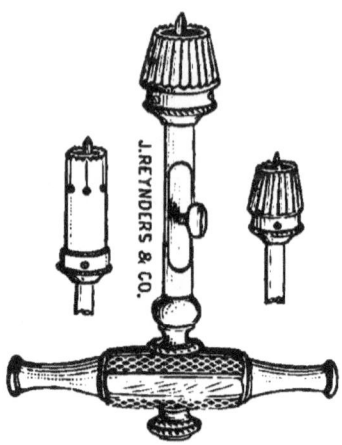

Fig. 148. Large conic Trephine on handle; small conic on right; cylindric on left.

Remedy.—Trephine; remove by trocar. But it is better to kill the animal as soon as it shows symptoms of the disease, and make the best of it.

HOOSE OR HUSK,

Scientifically known as verminous bronchitis, a parasitic disease of lambs and calves, is caused by a round worm (Strongylus filarius), which when mature resembles a piece of white thread. The female, which is larger than the male, is about $1\frac{1}{2}$ to 2 inches long. It inhabits the windpipe and bronchial tubes, but its embryos gain access to the deeper parts of the lungs, causing much irritation and patchy inflammation. The development of the worm is not understood. One thing, however, is certain—salt spread over the contaminated pastures is a preventive. Drainage is also useful. Destroy the lungs instead of feeding them to either people or cats. Cooking, however, kills the worms.

Many sheep suffering from hoose die from debility induced by diarrhea. Others die from suffocation, and many from congestion of the lungs, if exposed to a chill. Yellowish, millet-seed-like knots are found in the lungs of thousands of slaughtered sheep. They have often been mistaken for tubercle (consumption), but the microscope reveals the embryonic parasite in their interior.

Remedy.—Oil of turpentine, given in oil, milk, or lime water; it is still more prompt and effectual when injected into the trachea. Sulphurous or chlorine inhalations; spirit of chloroform, swallowed. Liberal, concentrated dietary. Isolate healthy sheep.

For doses, see pages 13 to 29.

ANOTHER WORM.

Another round worm, the twisted strongyle (Strongylus contortus), is often the cause of great loss among sheep. It is small, resembles a piece of red thread, and clings, by aid of barbs, to the membrane of the fourth stomach. It causes inflammation, diarrhea, wasting, and death. It is most seen on old pasture land, where there is plenty of fog for cover. Hence the necessity of removing the fog from such pastures by burning and by chain harrows. Top dressing with lime or salt should also be tried.

Remedy.—Chabert's oil, 1 part, oil turpentine, 3 parts. Kamala in doses of $\frac{1}{2}$ to 1 dram or more, given in thick gruel or molasses. Potassium picrate, 2 to 10 grains daily in linseed mucilage.

The only tapeworm of importance found in the sheep is the 'tænia expansa.' But it is questionable if it does much harm. It is seldom found unassociated with other parasites.

JOINT-ILL (ARTHRITIS),

Except as a purely sporadic disease, is due to a combination of two causes—(1) a depraved or impoverished condition of the mother's blood—nearly always, in my experience, brought about by injudicious management—whereby the milk contracts deleterious properties; (2) the combined effects of cold and wet. In some cases the actual cause is inflammation of the umbilical (navel) vein, as a result of which abscesses form in the liver. Suppurative inflammation of the joints follows. The probable primary cause of the disease is a micrococcus. (Walley.)

Lambs from two to five weeks old are very liable to the disorder. They are often stiff all over before the swellings appear. Sometimes they crawl on their knees. Sometimes they are prostrate. Usually they either die or become incurably lame and worthless.

Remedy.—Keep warm and dry. Mild purges if costive. Cordial medicine in hot gruel. Liniment: Oil of turpentine, 8 oz., strong solution of ammonia, 3 oz., soft soap, 4 oz.; digest, shake at intervals, adding water to make 2 quarts in all. Rub once or twice daily.

RHEUMATISM

Is the same in sheep as in other animals. Treat the same.

NAVEL-ILL OR NAVEL-POCKING

Is the result (1) of a depraved condition of the mother's system; (2) the action of poisonous germs on the clot of blood which is always found in the umbilical vein of newly born animals. If the system is healthy, no injury is caused by septic or poisonous organisms; otherwise the vitiated blood acts as pabulum for their development. Septic, sometimes erysipelatous, inflammation is set up, the products of which becoming absorbed, cause putrefactive inflammation of the joints, especially those of the hind limbs. In some cases, however, the inflammation extends along the cellular tissue to the fore legs in a forward direction and to the abdomen, thighs, and hind legs in a backward direction, the parts soon becoming of a black or purple hue from mortification.

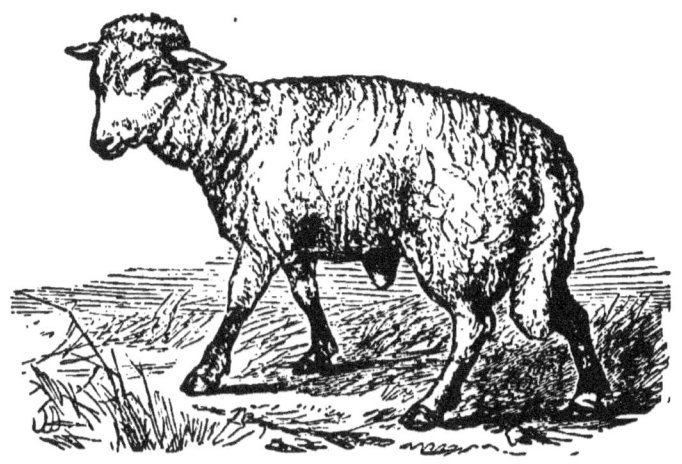

Fig. 148. Navel-Ill.

In both joint-ill and navel-ill the condition of the mother's blood should be improved, and the navel cord of the lamb should be tied with a silk or cotton ligature and dressed with an antiseptic lotion or liniment immediately after birth. (Walley.)

Aperients or neutral salts, such as sulphite or the salicylate of sodium, for ewes as well as lambs. Feed ewes very moderately.

LAMBING OR MILK FEVER (METRITIS),

Is probably caused by blood poisoning, blood poisoning being caused by germs called micrococci. The germs may be communicated from ewe to ewe by means of the blood on the hands of shepherds engaged in delivering ewes. Hence the necessity of disinfecting or washing the hands with 1 part of carbolic acid to 50 of water, or even with carbolic soap; or 3 grains permanganate of potassium to 1 oz. of water. The vagina of all infected ewes should also be washed, and the sick separated from the well. The disease is due sometimes perhaps to wounds and the retention and decomposition of the afterbirth.

Remedy.—Siphon or syringe uterus with tepid water or antiseptic. Remove remnants of placenta or blood clots; render any wounds aseptic (non-poisonous). Where walls of uterus are dilated or flaccid, inject solution of ergot and belladonna tincture. Rugs wrung out of hot water over loins and abdomen. Sulpho-carbolates, sulphites, hydronaphthol internally. If bowels are torpid, give half dose physic with ginger, gentian and molasses, and promote effect by laxative injections. Remove urine by catheter. Generous diet. Tonics, stimulants.

For doses, see pages 13 to 29.

ABORTION, AFTER-PAINS, AND GARGET

Are much the same in ewes as in cows. (See pages 289–291.) Ewes are more easily frightened than cows, and they are much oftener injured in casting. They should not be cast when pregnant, nor be roughly used. They should be carefully watched about the middle period of gestation. (The full period of gestation is about 150 days.) They should not be overfed and fattened just before lambing, for this is one of the chief causes of afterpains.

In garget (sore udder), 3 or 4 ounces of Epsom salt may be necessary, and may be repeated. Foment with warm water and rub with ointment, &c., as for cows.

LOUPING-ILL OR TREMBLING,

Says Williams, entails great loss among hill sheep every year. It has been described as a species of ergot intoxication or nervous excitement. There is sometimes squinting, at other times convulsive movements of the eyes.

There are also convulsive movements of the body and legs, and more or less increase of fluid in the spinal cord.

Veterinarians are not agreed as the cause of the disease, but as good food and pure water are preventives of it, bad food and impure water must be predisposing causes of it.

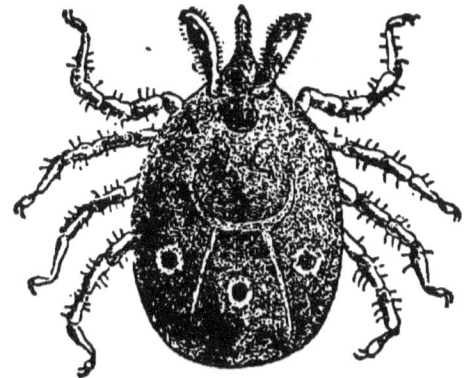

Fig. 149.   Sheep Tick.

Louping-ill is only seen on land infested with ticks. Ticks are the cause of the disease. It is possible, however, to have land infested with ticks and yet have sheep free of louping-ill, as all ticks do not seem to contain disease germs.

Improve moors and pastures where it exists. The cure is uncertain, but many sheep recover.

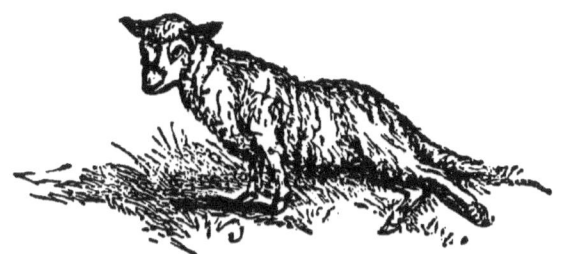

Fig. 150.   Louping-Ill or Hydro-Rachitis.

MEASLES

Which consists of red, irregular spots on the chest,

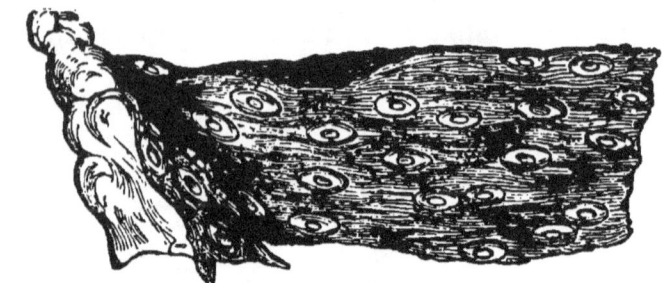

Fig. 151. Measles in pork.

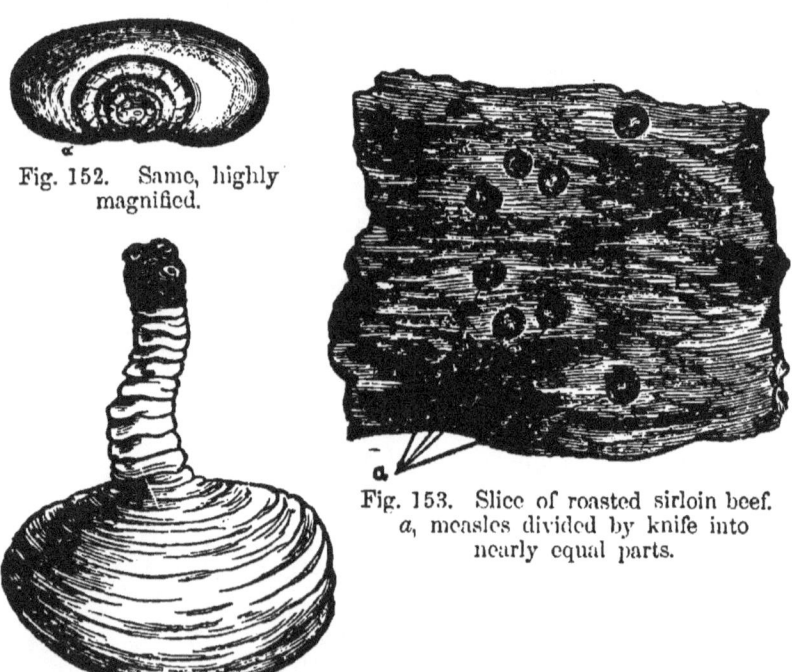

Fig. 152. Same, highly magnified.

Fig. 153. Slice of roasted sirloin beef. a, measles divided by knife into nearly equal parts.

Fig. 154. Measle or Bladder Worm of beef. Magnified.

thighs, head, and sides, is preceded by slight febrile symptoms, sneezing, coughing, swelling in the region of the head, discharge from the nostrils, hot mouth, dry skin, constipation, loss of appetite, &c. The skin has a peculiar odor. The red spots are hard in the center; if pressed, they appear white for a time. They seem to do good, for in about 24 hours after their appearance the febrile symptoms and swelling of the head subside. The spots become brownish in four or five days, and disappear in about five days more. The skin then peels off. Some symptoms of catarrh continue. In fatal cases diarrhea sets in about the ninth day.

We now know that mutton and beef as well as pork may become measled. These three kinds of measles are perfectly distinct from each other, and are derived from different species of tapeworm. (Williams.)

The disease can be transmitted by inoculation. Out of 103 animals inoculated by way of experiment, only 1 died.

Give plenty of water and niter to lick.

HOVEN

Is practically the same in sheep as in cattle (page 238).

Remedy.—Half a pint of linseed oil; if no relief follows in 2 or 3 hours, give ½ oz. aromatic spirit of ammonia in a pint of warm water, or about 6 oz. of brandy

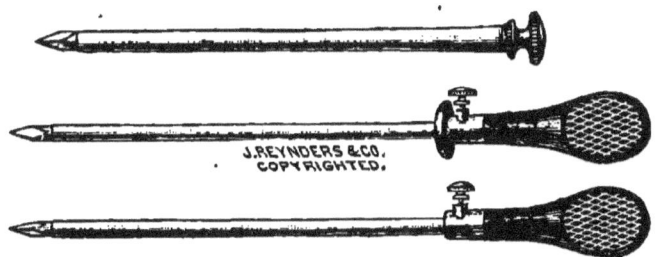

Fig. 155. Trocars.

or whisky, slightly diluted with warm water. Trocar if necessary, and retain canula as long as there are signs of distress.

TETANUS (LOCK-JAW),

Is about the same in sheep as in horses and cattle, and should be treated the same. The animal may die in twelve hours. Exposure to cold, especially after shearing, is conducive of the disease.

Keep warm and quiet. Give gruel, to which add a little gin. Castor oil or Epsom salt; repeated if necessary. (See pages 53 and 234.)

RABIES

Kills sheep in from three to seven weeks. It develops itself in from two to four weeks after the bite, but it may remain dormant till the eleventh week. The sheep gradually grow sick. Sometimes they die of paralysis, at

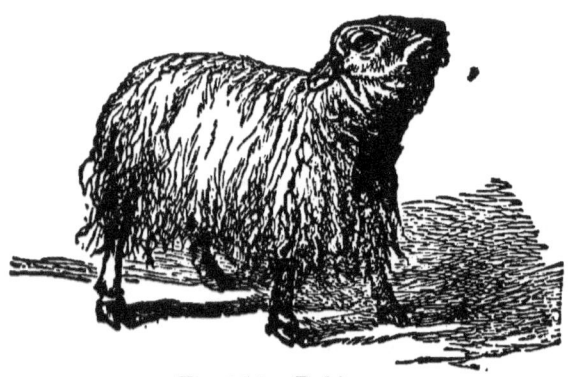

Fig. 156. Rabies.

other times of convulsions. They have great thirst, but no fear of water; become furious and fight among themselves, but do not bite mankind. (See page 50.)

SHEEP BOT-FLIES

Are a little larger than ordinary house-flies. They are of an ashy gray color. They deposit their eggs in the nostrils of sheep during July and August, where, if not expelled, they remain till spring. Being then full-grown, they fall to the ground and become pupæ. The pupæ-cases open in summer and they are freed. They deposit their eggs and live till fall. The maggots penetrate to the sinuses and sometimes even to the brain.

Remedy.—Snuff, solution of common salt, tobacco infusion, diluted vinegar, or a weak solution of turpentine may be injected into the nose. Many flies will be expelled by sneezing. If any remain in the sinuses, trephine and syringe with tepid water containing a small proportion of carbolic acid.

RED WATER

Kills sheep and lambs as well as cattle. (See page 270.) If the disease is discovered in time, slaughter for food. It is claimed that the disease is due to a lack of iron in the system. Whether true or not, salt of iron seems to be useful. Give 15 grains of sulphate of iron.

OPHTHALMIA (Inflamed Eyes),

Is frequent and sometimes severe in sheep. As a rule it is the same as in the horse (page 136), but it has special features. One of these is where the eyelids adhere to the eyeball, common but not confined to sheep suffering with scab. Shepherds separate the lid from the ball by means of a thin, hard, and polished piece of wood, wash with a decoction of mallows or poppyheads, and sometimes rub in a little oil.

Sometimes the disease is epizootic—among cattle as well as sheep. This form is known as 'the blind,' and is peculiar to young sheep, especially when exposed. It is dangerous, besides which the blind animal is liable to fall over a precipice. Apparently it is due to exposure to cold, but it may possibly be due to a micro-organism. It is highly infectious.

Remedy.—Dark, well ventilated shed; nutritious food, with a lump of rock salt in trough. Tar or ointment of salicylic acid around margin of eye, renewed in four days. Rub with a mixture of castor oil and corrosive sublimate, or blow, with quill, salt dried by heating into the eye.

In diseases of the eyes, in either sheep or cattle, it is better, when practicable, to fatten and slaughter than to waste time and money in treatment, especially in such diseases as amaurosis (glass-eye), glaucoma, &c.

NON-SECRETION OF MILK (AGALACTIA),

When not depending on any disease nor on wasting of the udder, may usually be restored, or partially restored, by the use of nutritious food and the following draft: Powdered aniseed, 2 oz., powdered gentian, 2 oz., in a pint of warm water or beer, 2 or 3 times daily.

The ears of sheep require to be kept clean, as they are liable to inflammation from dirt and maggots. The head is carried lower than usual, often a little to one side, and is occasionally shaken.

Fractured and Broken Limbs are sometimes curable, but unless the sheep is very valuable, it is cheaper to slaughter.

PART IV.

THE DISEASES OF SWINE.

THE stomach and digestive organs of swine and dogs, says Dun, much resemble those of man and are acted on in nearly the same way by most drugs. The best purge for swine is three or four ounces of Epsom salt, or a like quantity of linseed or castor oil, given in a shallow spoon or bottle. An assistant should hold the animal firmly by the ears. From two to five drams of aloes is also a good purge, but it takes from twelve to fifteen hours to operate. Also one to three drams of jalap, but large doses may cause nausea or even vomiting. Five to ten drops of croton oil is a prompt and effectual drastic purge, but requires, as in most other patients, to be used with much caution.

To be healthy, swine (in herds) should be kept in large fields or inclosures, and be provided with grass, pure, running water, and shade, especially in summer. Corn and other fattening foods are good for winter. Careful feeding, breeding, and management are very important factors in swine rearing, more important perhaps than all the medicines combined. Still simple disorders may be successfully treated.

Unlike cattle and sheep, the pig has but one stomach, which is nearly as simple in structure as that of the horse. Its teeth are adapted to the mastication of many kinds of food. The tushes are formidable weapons.

SWINE PLAGUE OR SWINE ANTHRAX,

Also known as hog cholera, red soldier, blue sickness, measles, erysipelas, intestinal fever, typhoid fever, &c., is a highly contagious and infective disease. It has a period of incubation, after inoculation, of about five days, when the temperature is 104 or 106°, succeeded by signs of general ill health and usually a rash on the skin. It is epizootic, and is the most fatal swine disease. Pigs dif-

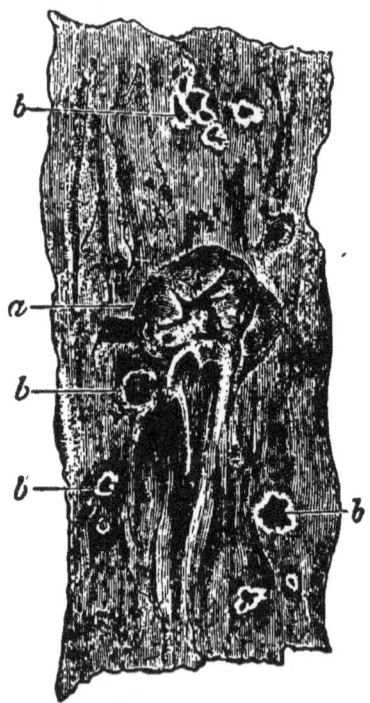

Fig. 157. Part of cæcum (blind gut). *a*, ilio-cæcal opening. *b, b, b,* ulcers in various stages.

fer in their susceptibility to it. It appears to be caused by contagion or infection only, no amount of mismanagement, filth, lack of drainage, or decomposing food being sufficient to induce it. (Williams.)

Symptoms.—Loss of appetite; general prostration; small and frequent pulse; hanging ears; sullen appearance; painful and haggard expression; watery eyes, the conjunctive membranes being red and spotted; dirty secretion about the eyelids, usually preceded by a red blush and red spots on the ears, the abdomen, and internal aspects of the extremities. The reddened spots are at first hot and painful to the touch, but become cold, humid, and insensible even to the pricking of a pin. As the disease advances trembling and convulsions are manifested; grinds the teeth; flexor muscles of limbs contract; stands on toes. These symptoms are succeeded by paralysis of the posterior extremities, or of the whole body, involuntary defacation (bowel evacuation), and high colored and even bloody urine. The bowels are at first generally torpid, but the feces may be soft and mixed with very black, fetid blood and thick, tenacious mucus. Diarrhea, however, often sets in; the evacuations are then profuse and exhaustive; the breathing becomes catching and convulsive; a painful cough is present; the convulsions increase in violence and may continue to do so till the end; but sometimes the animal becomes comatose and remains so till the end.

In some cases the first observable symptoms remain stationary from 24 to 48 hours; then the surface of the body becomes burning hot and very sensitive to the touch, notably at the sides and abdominal walls. If touched, the animal cries with pain. To these signs are added trembling, convulsions, grinding of the teeth, and tetanic (tetanus or lock-jaw-like) contraction of the muscles, succeeded by rapid diminution of temperature. The membranes of the eyes become brown, the eyes themselves bleared; tongue dirty, thick, bluish; the animal, extended on its litter, is incapable of any regulated movement, and dies in from 24 to 48 hours.

These symptoms are liable to various modifications, depending on the intensity of the fever and the locality of the poison. In some cases the virus seems to expend itself on the serous membranes, causing either inflammation of the peritoneum or pleurisy; sometimes on the mucous membranes, as shown by bronchitis or bronchopneumonic congestion and hemorrhage, and enteric (intestinal) congestion and ulceration; sometimes even to perforation or rupture of the bowel.

In many cases the animal is amaurotic; wanders to and fro; falls, rolls, kicks. Now and then it will rise from its bed and give a piercing cry, the whole body being involuntarily convulsed. (Williams.)

Dr. H. J. Ditmers says swine plague "is not a single or separate disease, but rather a group of several kindred diseases, similar to each other in regard to causes, morbid process, contagiousness, and final termination, but differing very much as to symptoms, seat of morbid process, course, and duration."

Swine plague is classed among the incurable diseases.

APOPLEXY

Occurs usually in fat hogs. Several forms have been described, but all are chiefly caused perhaps by too much blood and confinement—lack of exercise. The specific blood poison of anthrax may not be present. The diseases of pigs to which the term apoplexy is applied, however, partake more of the nature of anthrax than otherwise, especielly in young and growing animals.

Symptoms.—Restlessness; eyes bloodshot; appetite variable; constipation; dung and urine scanty. As the animal eats, it suddenly stops, reels, and falls down dead, a great quantity of foam issuing from the mouth.

Remedy.—As apoplexy is a most fatal complaint, prompt preventive measures should be instituted on its first appearance. Place healthy swine on a low diet; exercise; cleanliness. Give Epsom salt, 2 to 4 oz., calomel, 3 to 10 grains, ginger, 2 to 3 drams, with molasses and linseed mucilage in proportion—immediately. Give same dose to sick hog, that is, if it does not die too soon. Clysters for constipation. When down and breathing heavily, bleed from the veins of the inner surface of the ears. The palate veins and also those of the fore limbs may be opened if necessary.

EPILEPSY

Prevails more among swine than among either cattle or sheep. Its exact nature is not understood further than that it depends on some peculiar morbid condition of the nervous system, probably degeneration of tissue, arising from defective nutrition; also on remote causes, such as abscesses, tumors, &c., in the spleen, brain, and other organs; worms in the stomach or intestines, and other conditions producing reflex action. It is peculiar to young animals generally, but it occurs in the old also as a result of blood diseases, blood poisoning, &c. It is rarely curable.

Symptoms.—Severe convulsions, with coma (sleepiness) and foaming at the mouth; staggers; eyes protrude and

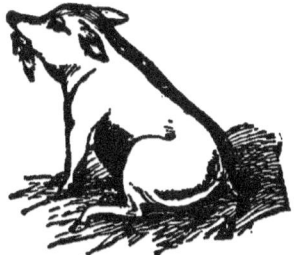

Fig. 158. Epilepsy.

stare; violent champing of teeth; drops on haunches; fore limbs rigid; head elevated, turned from side to side rapidly and now and then tossed up; muscles convulsed; urine and feces pass involuntarily; tongue bitten; falls, struggles violently, and soon becomes unconscious; heart beats strong; membranes increased in color. A long sleep may follow, or the animal may soon regain consciousness, but only to be speedily reattacked; dies.

Remedy.—If caused by nervous disorder, give belladonna or atrophine. If from worms, give a vermifuge. Proper food and housing; exercise. At the time of attack little can be done. Dashing cold water over the head and face is the most proper course, deferring other measures till the seizure has passed. Strychnine, quassia, gentian or other tonic for lack of blood; less nutritious diet for too much blood; also exercise. As a means of reducing the severity of an attack, and while there is power to swallow, chloroform, chloric or sulphuric ether, chloral hydrate, &c., should be given, or the animal may inhale the first, the latter being injected beneath the skin. When it is known that a nerve is at fault, it may be divided, or the firing-iron may be applied over the locality.

For doses, see pages 13 to 29.

TRICHINA SPIRALIS (WORMS),

According to Williams, is usually found within capsules or cysts, occupying the muscles of some animals, such as the pig, or even of man. When full-grown, the female is much larger than the male, being one-eighth and one-eighteenth of an inch in length respectively.

Small animals, such as rats, cats, and rabbits, when seriously infected, like man, soon succumb to the disease. The health of larger animals, however, is rarely affected. A pig that was experimented on in the Royal Veterinary College, showed no signs of the disease, notwithstanding an after-death examination indicated that its flesh probably contained 16,000,000 of living worms! Other pigs, however, showed much general disturbance and suffering, arising from the irritation of the worms in the intestines and during their passage into the muscular tissue. The irritation of the alimentary canal, which lessens toward the end of the first week after pigs have swallowed trichinæ, is denoted by loss of appetite, vomiting, colic, diarrhea, dullness, arching of the back, and an inclination to lie down and hide in the litter. These symptoms, except the diarrhea, usually disappear in from six to eight days.

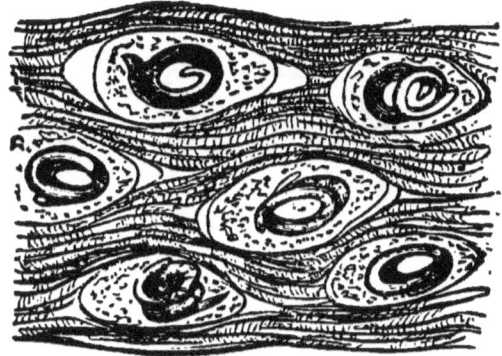

Fig. 159. Pork Flesh Worm (Trichina Spiralis), imbedded in the flesh.

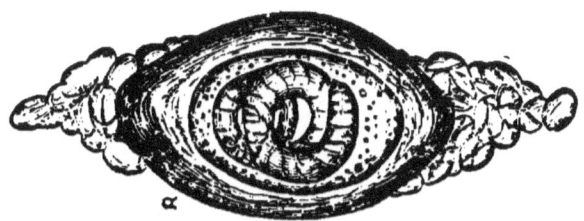

Fig. 160. The immature worm, highly magnified.

When the trichinæ are numerous, the membranous passage of a great number of them induce in some pigs a fatal inflammation of the peritoneum: in others a form of inflammation of the intestines, with ejection of false membrane.

Trichinous pork, if used at all, must be well cooked. Great heat is necessary to kill all the worms. The only safe plan is to cook *all* pork meat thoroughly.

328   THE DISEASES OF SWINE.

MEASLES

In swine, cattle, or sheep means an internal or intramuscular disorder, not an external eruptive disease. It

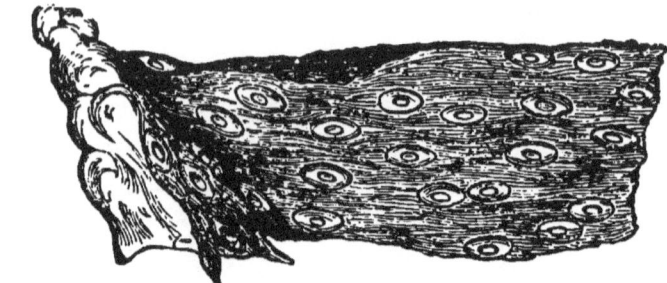

Fig. 161.   Measles in pork.

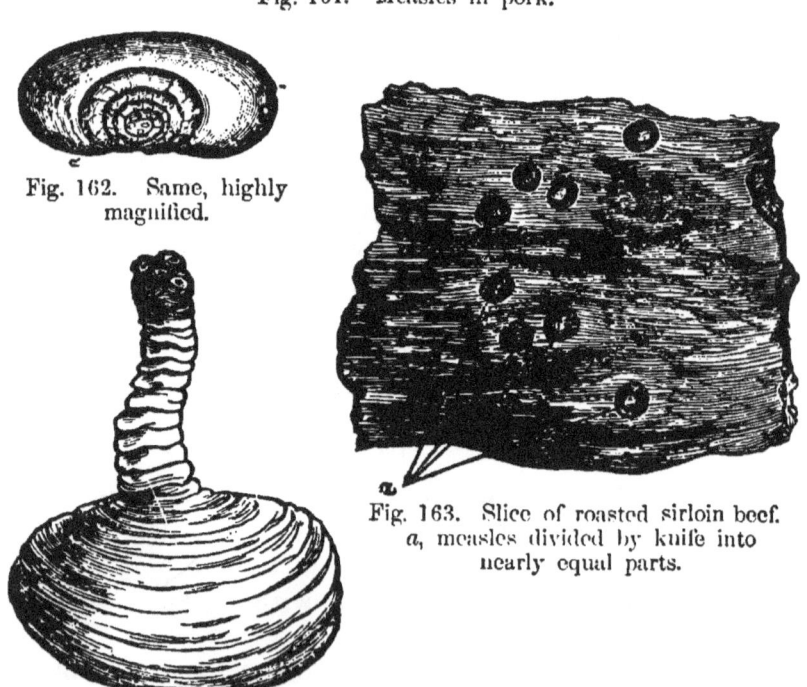

Fig. 162.   Same, highly magnified.

Fig. 163.   Slice of roasted sirloin beef. *a*, measles divided by knife into nearly equal parts.

Fig. 164.   Measle or Bladder Worm of beef.   Magnified.

is caused by a tapeworm technically known as 'Tænia solium' (solitary tapeworm), which imbeds itself in the flesh. The eggs of the worm are taken up by the pig in its search for food here and there, especially among dung heaps and other filth. The worm is nearly spheroidal in shape, having an average diameter of about 1-694th of an inch, and therefore readily enters the circulation, whence it is carried to various parts of the body. It is very prolific. It lives about two years and produces at least 1,600 joints, each of which contains 53,000 eggs—total, 85,000,-000. Fortunately, like the ova of other parasites, many are destroyed in various ways.

After the ova enter the flesh, several changes occur. The germs are inclosed in small cysts or bladders, each

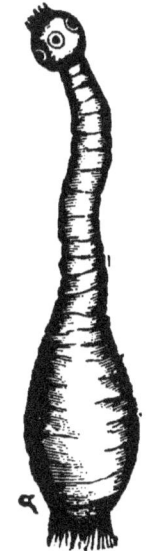 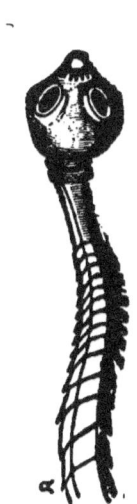

Fig. 165. Larva of Pork Tapeworm, with caudal vesicle, liberated from cyst. Hooks at top.

Fig. 166. Head of Tænia Solium or Pork Tapeworm.

having a small, rudimentary head, with hooks and suckers, &c. They remain in the body till the pig is slaughtered, when, if the pork is not thoroughly cooked, they produce full-grown tapeworms. An unusually large number of them may kill a hog. They are peculiar to the tender flesh of young animals, being unable to enter the solid flesh of those even one year old. (Armitage.)

Prevention.—Feed swine on healthy food.

PROTRUSION OF THE RECTUM

Is common. The causes are violent straining during constipation, diarrhea, impaction of the stomach, worms, piles, and injuries inflicted in the anus or intestine; it may also follow difficult parturition and stitching across the vulva to prevent eversion of the uterus or bladder.

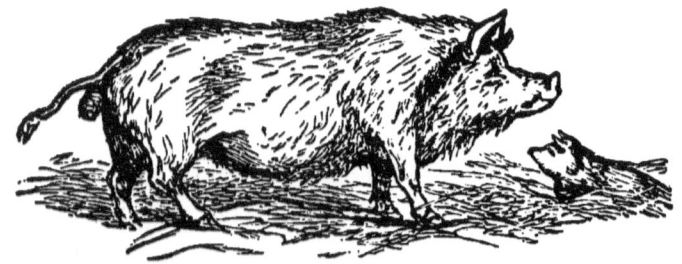

Fig. 167. Protrusion of the Rectum.

Remedy.—When recent, the color bright, and the tumor of moderate dimensions, merely wash parts gently with warm water, the whole carefully compressed at the sides by the fingers, which are spread so as to include as much of the tumor as possible. By a kneading movement, in which the thumbs should be especially active, the central part gradually returns, followed by the outer, until the whole is replaced. Subsequent straining is to be checked—when not caused by constipation—by a full dose of opium or chloroform, chloric ether, &c., and injections of the same fluids may be required. When constipation is the cause, purgatives should be given, combined with anodynes. Change food if necessary. Sometimes the organ is protruded six or seven inches, is greatly swollen, and now and then lacerated by being seized by other pigs. Foment for two hours or more, and if necessary apply ice, astringents, &c. In other cases, when time has elapsed, the organ may be livid or dark purple in color and injured by the movements of the patient. Treat as above and recovery often follows. The cause of the protrusion must be ascertained and removed before a permanent cure can be effected. (Armitage.)

CONSTIPATION

Is caused by the excessive use of highly stimulating food and lack of exercise.

Symptoms.—Dull; refuses food; avoids companions, even hiding in the straw or in a dark corner of the stye; is obstinate, even bearing punishment before rising; walks crampy, grunting or screaming; anus clean and firmly contracted; belly tender, pressure on which causing the animal to scream, rush away, and crouch at a distance;

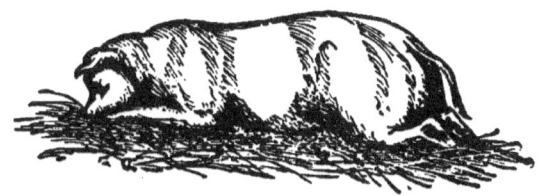

Fig. 168. Usual position when suffering from Constipation

the invariable position is as shown above (Fig. 168); pulse rapid, full, hard; membranes injected; abdominal pain; up and down, screaming or grunting; urine deficient, high colored, ammoniacal. If not relieved, the symptoms increase in severity; becomes frantic; apoplexy may end life. Sometimes the abdominal pains increase, diarrhea ensues, and the animal dies in from 12 to 24 hours of prostration.

Remedy.—Purge early with Epsom salt, 2 to 4 oz., powdered ginger, 1 dram, powdered gentian, 2 drams, calomel, 5 to 10 grains, mixed in linseed mucilage. Injections of soap and warm water every half hour. In 2 hours after giving the internal dose, give the following stimulant: Spirit nitric ether, 2 to 4 drams, essence of ginger, ½ dram, tincture of belladonna, 1 dram, in a half pint of warm linseed tea. Friction to skin; general comfort. Laxative food at first, in sparing quantities and at regular intervals. Drink, tepid water, with a small quantity of oatmeal, linseed tea, &c. Let animal roam. Careful attention to food to prevent another attack. (Armitage.)

SCROTAL RUPTURE (HERNIA),

Is very common among young pigs, and such should be castrated by the covered operation. The general practice is to castrate in the usual way and stitch the divided scrotum. Sometimes castrators include the intestine in the suture, causing death. I have cut pigs with hernia by merely inclosing the scrotum in a loop of twine—first returning the intestine—and allowing the parts to be removed by sloughing; and they have done well. Pigs are peculiarly liable, during some seasons, to suffer from tetanus (so-called lock-jaw) after castration. (Williams.)

CATARRH

Is the same in nature in swine as in other animals, and should be treated the same. Give laxatives in warm mashes, and protect from exposure to cold, dampness, and drafts. (See pages 70 and 258.)

DIARRHEA,

Which usually attacks sucking pigs, should be treated on the same general principles as diarrhea in other animals. The dose must be small for young pigs, and is best given in a shallow spoon or bottle, but for older animals it may be mixed in a dainty dish. In sucking pigs see that the sow has healthy food; in fact, look to the food in every case. (See pages 107, 246).

PARALYSIS OF HIND QUARTERS

Is not common, but it should be combated with care and suitable remedies. Simple turpentine rubbed over the loins and back sometimes gives relief. If it fails, rub with the following penetrating liniment: Alcohol, 1 pint, ammonia, ¼ oz., oil organum, ½ oz., oil sassafras, ½ oz., tincture opium, ¼ oz., tincture capsicum, ½ oz., oil turpentine, ½ oz., camphor, ¼ oz. A teaspoonful of this liniment, diluted with a wine-glass of water, will check diarrhea or colic in man as well as the lower animals. Repeat dose if necessary. Horses and cattle would require about ½ an oz. internally for colic; water in proportion.

RHEUMATISM

Should be treated with the above liniment, or some other equally soothing and penetrating. Give gentle laxative in food if necessary, and keep swine in warm, dry quarters.

INFLAMMATION OF THE LUNGS (PNEUMONIA),

Also called heaves, thumps, &c., is a dangerous and usually incurable disease. (See pages 79, 261.)

QUINSY

Is an inflammation of the throat and adjacent parts, accompanied by more or less fever. It is similar to if not the same as laryngitis (sore throat). Apply warm fomentations and rub with soothing liniments. If external suppuration takes place, encourage it, and treat it as a boil. If the animal can swallow, a tablespoonful of turpentine and oil may be given in swill.

Quinsy, or strangles, as it is sometimes called, on account perhaps of the difficulty of breathing, is a dangerous disease.

MANGE

Is caused by the mite illustrated below (Fig. 169). It is transmissible to man. (See pages 168, 281, 301.)

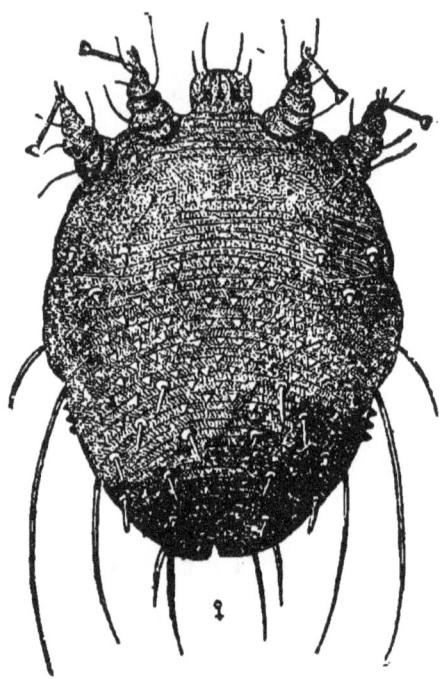

Fig. 169. The mite or acarus known as Sarcoptes suis. Magnified.

For **Lice,** see pages 168, 284.

For **Jaundice,** see pages 133, 253.

For **Foot and Mouth Disease,** see page 224.

For **Scrofula or Tuberculosis,** see pages 91, 225.

EVERYBODY'S PAINT-BOOK

IS THE TITLE OF A NEW WORK ON

INDOOR AND OUTDOOR PAINTING,

Which should find a place in EVERY HOUSEHOLD in the land. It is designed to teach people how they may DO THEIR OWN PAINTING and save the expense of a professional painter. Full directions for mixing and applying paints are given. It also tells all about VARNISHING, POLISHING, STAINING, PAPER-HANGING, KALSOMINING, etc., as well as how to RENOVATE FURNITURE so that it will look as good as new. It tells all about HOUSE CLEANING and putting things to rights so far as they can be done by Paint and Kalsomine. Many useful hints on ARTISTIC WORK for HOME DECORATION are given.

PAINTING FARM IMPLEMENTS.

Full directions are given for painting all kinds of farm implements, with a list of best colors to use.

CLEANING HOUSE.
Under this head full directions are given for mixing and applying kalsomine to ceilings and walls. It also tells how to make and use stencils for ornamenting ceilings. Gives detailed directions for paper-hanging, so that every one can paper a room successfully. Tells how to make damask walls, etc. Tells how to paint a kitchen or chamber floor, varnish oil-cloth, paint the front door, varnish rustic work, restore chromos and oil paintings, renovate picture frames, clean marble, etc.

PAINTING OUTBUILDINGS.
Full directions are given for mixing and applying paint to outbuildings, fences, etc.

PAINTING ROOFS.
Tells how to paint both tin and shingle roofs, and what roofs are most durable.

PAINTING FARM WAGONS.
Complete directions for painting farm wagons are given, including mixing and the colors best to use.

CARRIAGE PAINTING.
Precise and detailed directions for painting buggies and carriages, showing each step in the work, are given.

HOME DECORATIONS.
Under this head full directions for making the beautiful and popular SPATTER WORK are given. Ladies take great delight in this work, and many beautiful pictures can be made.

It tells how to Polish a Piano or Organ, how to imitate Ground Glass, how to make paint for Black-Boards, Stain for Oak Graining, Mahogany Stain, Rosewood Stain, etc. Also tells about Gilding, Bronzing, Silvering, and Lacquering.

The book contains a large number of illustrations, and is handsomely bound in extra cloth, with ink and gold, and will be sent to any part of the country on receipt of price $1.00. Agents wanted. Address

M. T. RICHARDSON, Publisher,
84 and 86 READE ST., NEW YORK.

$1000 Worth of Law for $1.50

"How to be Your Own Lawyer" is the title of an entirely new book of over 500 pages, adapted for use in every State and Territory in the Union, and is by far the best and most complete work of the kind ever published. It gives instruction on all the most important law points which a **Farmer, Mechanic, Merchant**, or anybody else would want to know about, and if carefully studied and kept at hand for consultation when needed will **save any man**, in the course of an ordinary business career, hundreds, if not thousands of dollars. It is a lawyer whose retaining fee (the price of the book $1.50) has to be paid but **once in a life-time.** Plain and concise directions are given and forms furnished for the transaction of all kinds of business, and the preparation of every description of legal document in common use, such as Agreements, Bonds, Deeds, Leases, Notes, Mortgages, Wills, Etc. It takes up and treats in alphabetical order over 70 different subjects, as follows: Acknowledgment and Proof of Deeds, Administrators, Affidavits, Agents, Agreements, Apprentices, Arbitration, Assignments, Auctions, Bankruptcy, Bills of Sale, Bonds, Bills of Exchange, Cattle and Dog Laws, Collection of Debts, Common Carriers, Consideration, Contracts, Copyright, Corporate Associations, Custom House, Deeds, Divorce, Dower, Drafts, Executors, Exemption Laws, Farmers, Fences, Guaranty, Guardian and Ward, Highways, Hotels and Boarding-Houses, Husband and Wife, Insolvency, Insurance (Life, Fire, and Marine), Interest, Internal Revenue, Landlord and Tenant, Law of Place, Leases, Letters of Credit, Letter-Writing, Libel, Slander, Licenses, Lien Laws Limitation of Actions, Marriage, Master and Servant, Mining Laws, Minor, Mortgages, Naturalization, Pensions, Parent and Child, Parliamentary Rules, Partnership, Patents, Payment and Tender, Personal Property, Partition, Power of Attorney, Promissory Notes, Real Estate, Receipts and Releases, Rights of Married Women, Schools, Shipping, Subscription Papers (How to Draw), Trade-Marks, Trespass, Trusts and Trustees, Vessels, Voters, Wills, Warranty of Horses.

There is also a very complete Dictionary of Legal Terms; Tables for the Computation of Interest; Measurement of LAND, LUMBER, LOGS, GRAIN; Legal Weight of a Bushel of Grain, Seed, and Roots; Quantity of Seed required to plant an Acre; Table showing Paper Required to make a Book of any Size; U. S. Land Measure; Number of Brick Required to Construct any building; Presidential Vote from 1824 to 1885; Time for holding Elections in different States; Population of the U. S.; Prices of various Commodities for fifty-three years; Valuable Rules for the use of Farmers and Mechanics; and much other important information. A copy of this valuable work, handsomely bound in extra cloth, with ink side-stamp, will be mailed to any address on receipt of $1.50. Address

M. T. RICHARDSON, Publisher,

84 and 86 Reade Street, New York.

www.ingramcontent.com/pod-product-compliance
Lightning Source LLC
Chambersburg PA
CBHW021213240426
43667CB00038B/362